I CAN'T SAVE YOU

I CAN'T
SAVE YOU

A MEMOIR

Anthony Chin-Quee

RIVERHEAD BOOKS • NEW YORK • 2023

RIVERHEAD BOOKS
An imprint of Penguin Random House LLC
penguinrandomhouse.com

Library of Congress Cataloging-in-Publication Data

LIBRARY OF CONGRESS CONTROL NUMBER: 2022039768
ISBN 9780593418888 (hardcover)
ISBN 9780593418901 (ebook)

Printed in the United States of America
1st Printing

Book design by Amanda Dewey

For Pippa:

*I'm able to love you so easily and completely
only because I learned to love myself before you arrived.*

Thank you for choosing me.

Author's Note

The idea of a memoir is fascinating to me. Its very fancy French etymology defines it as an account of an author's own mémoires—their memories. But here's the thing about memories: they are informed by one's state of mind, both in the past when they were formed and in the present as they're being told. With that said, all events depicted in this book are as true as my memory has allowed them to be.

The only intentionally falsified portions of this story are the names and identifying details of some individuals I've shared my life with. Their stories, experiences, and perspectives are not mine to tell, so I have done my best to respect their privacy by obscuring some personal details of the innocent and not-so-innocent.

All of this is to say thank you in advance. For being here. For reading and for listening to the truths that took me a lifetime to find. The opportunity to put this story into your hands has been an immeasurable gift to me.

Hold on to your butts. It's a wild ride.

—Tony

Contents

I CAN'T SAVE YOU

Prologue

I know you hate me.

You only had to say it once, but I believed you.

Because you'd never hated anything before. And nothing since.

You turn yourself inside out to forgive and accept everything and everyone.

Except for me.

And I get it. I was never able to lead you to the perfection you thought would mend you.

But I kept pushing. I kept appealing, encouraging, pleading to the parts of you that could be amazing if only you'd let them try, fail, be forgiven, and try again.

But you hear failure louder than any voice.

So you locked me away in the space between dreaming and waking, where you could write me off as an echo of whatever story you'd told yourself overnight.

And that's fine. I was built for patience—the trait that always drove you nuts about me, especially when I got preachy about it.

But something's not right. Lately my attempts at patience only leave me squirming restlessly. My diminished voice—the one that fell into disrepair once you chose to become deaf to my calls—has been croaking desperately back to life. I've been propelled by an urgency, and I've only just understood its origin: fear.

Fear of time.

Suddenly I don't think we have enough of it left.

So that's why I've crawled my way up to the surface now. That's why I'm screaming with every shade of voice you've left me.

You're in danger. You're teetering on the edge of something tragic.

Please let me in. Together we can save you.

You just need to wake the fuck up.

CHIN-QUEE, M.D.

So, I had the dream again.

The Vegas dream, where I wake up in a hotel room face-to-face with my father.

I still can't tell how old he is. Or how he got there. His ever-present glasses are nowhere to be found. Neither are mine. Maybe that's why his face is so hard to read. Not hard to see—hard to *understand*. He still looks way too much like me. Far more than in real life, but I guess my sleeping brain fucks with genetics way more than I do in the daylight.

And still, just like all of the other times this dream has found me, he doesn't say a word. Nothing but silence from my old man as he studies me with eyes that are just a *little* too much like mine.

Then he smiles.

And I wake up screaming.

Heart pounding against my ribs, sweating bullets, arms and legs thrashing, the whole thing.

It definitely freaked out the chick who was sleeping next to me.

I tried to apologize, but she was already fumbling in the dark for her clothes. She'd forgotten: she had some place to be at (*checks analog watch in the dark*) 3:15 a.m. On a Sunday. I can admit I was moderately bummed that she didn't even ask if I was okay. But honestly, we'd only just met last night in a hookah bar. Hadn't quite reached the *I'll-be-your-late-night-dream-trauma-therapist* stage of the relationship. Lucky for her I didn't add insult to injury by peeing the bed. That's actually been happening a lot lately. And by "a lot" I mean more than never, which is way too often for a fucking grown man with a medical degree. So run, Carrie or Courtney or Carney or whatever your goddamn name was. Run for your life and don't look back. You definitely dodged a bullet.

What I'm saying is, I think I might be fucked.

I think my brain is . . . short-circuiting? Inhospitable? Broken? Melting out through my ears? Goddamn it, none of those feel right. What I'm trying to say is I feel . . . asphyxiated, I think? Like there's a vise around every muscle in my body and every corner of my mind and with every twitch or stretch or idea or hope the crank spins and the jaws squeeze tighter and nothing anywhere can breathe.

And that's a run-on sentence. With a mediocre mix of metaphors that've been stretched within an inch of their lives. Great start.

I suppose what I should lead with is the infuriating truth: I'm not good with words. Actually, I *am* really good with *some* words. I can bullshit my way through just about any situation that I don't deem personally consequential with the charisma to make anyone believe me. It's just one of the gifts that make me so deceptively toxic. But I'm very, highly . . . ungood at the other words. The ones that matter. To me.

Selective mutism. And I don't just throw the phrase around to flex SAT-level vocab retention—I'm pretty sure it's been baked into my faulty brain wiring since I first blinked and breathed. There were countless times before I even had a tenth birthday when I found myself consumed by feelings that weren't as simple as the ones I'd learned in school. You remember those books we used to read in class: point to the colorful cartoon faces whose entire existence demanded they live up to the name *Happy! Sad! Angry! Scared!* Never any faces for their more complicated descendants *Guilty! Traumatized! Ashamed! Inadequate! Depressed!* And even if they'd considered expanding the feelings family tree, I don't think the illustrators would have had the guts to draw the deeper truth: all of those new emotions would most likely wear the same expression as the unassuming, flat-mouthed pastel disembodied head named *Fine! Yeah, Everything's Fine!*

And so the result was a seven-year-old boy who appeared totally fine. Until he started going to sleepover parties at perfectly nice children's houses only to knock on their parents' bedroom doors at 11:00 p.m., tearfully pleading to go home. He'd sit in a choke hold of wordless responses to his father's frenzied demands that he explain himself, and accept the blame for wasting gas and precious night hours that should belong to sleep. And then he'd be fine again for weeks. Maybe months. Until he fell uncharacteristically quiet for a few days, then plunged into a fevered, vomiting illness for a few more, only to miraculously recover when his report card arrived with nothing but "exceeds expectations" in all subjects. His psychologist mother was no fool, and she did her professional best to poke and prod for the meaning behind his clearly psychosomatic freak-out, but to no avail. Because words are hard. And truthful words are even harder.

Where does a kid find the words to explain that the sleepover party debacle wasn't just homesickness but also an all-consuming, unfounded dread that something terrible would happen to his family if he wasn't home to know everyone was asleep and safe? Or that he'd been caught doodling in a notebook at school one day, sending him down a spiral of panic that he'd not only fail his classes but also be expelled from school and earn the rare honor of a belt-assisted ass whupping on the living room floor, and so the panic shut his body down, rendering it defenseless and susceptible to whatever opportunistic infections waited to fuck up insolent children?

Way, *way* too many words.

And even if the words had existed for me, I still wouldn't have said them aloud. Because I'd somehow always had it in my head that my fears were faults, and faults were failures. And if I was a failure, who would want me?

That's not normal, right? Like I said: faulty brain wiring.

My sputtering mind came equipped with a pressure release valve—one with a mercifully low word-count requirement. I've always found it easy to make things. Imagine things. Mold all of the abstract, slippery things into shapes and sounds and movements and characters that would say so much more than I could say. Art, I believe it's called.

Back when I was first learning to swallow the pain of asking for things my family couldn't afford, I started drawing my own comics. I had several marbled composition notebooks full of the serialized adventures of a too-cool-for-school, wrap-around-sunglasses-toting, Rollerblading kid from Brooklyn who solved low-stakes neighborhood crimes with the assistance of the unique powers of his Rollerblades. He'd then hold celebratory press conferences where he thanked his Rollerblades, without which justice would not and could not have been done. Any guesses as to what I was too scared to put on my Christmas list that year?

And oh, man, music—a language that always made sense to me. I grew up in the days before music streaming. Pre–MP3 player. Actually, pre-internet. I'm talking about the time when FM radio ruled pop culture, and your parents had record players with big-ass floor speakers, and when personal cassette tape players were the height of luxury until your nonrechargeable batteries bit the dust after two hours. Unlike today, music was not available everywhere all the time back then. So I carried it with me in my bones. Without saying a word, I'd converse with melodies all day, bounce along to syncopated, jazzy drumbeats with each footstep, and hold out hope that I'd stumble across an F major 9 or B-flat major 7 chord hidden in a radio pop song. At the time, I didn't know how or why the notes fit together so beautifully. All I knew was that they'd reliably send literal waves of euphoria through my body. Probably not on the spectrum of normal responses to hearing DMX or the Backstreet Boys, but at least my weirdo brain synapses were good for something.

I went on to play a few instruments, and I think that any time I touched my saxophone or piano keys or drumsticks I did so in search of those fleeting moments of joyful clarity—when, in the space of a single breath, a collection of dancing notes would soothe the anxiety crackling in my muscles and tickle my messy subconscious feelings until their heads popped out, just long enough for a momentary bashful wink, gone before I could see their faces.

Oh, and movies! And not just watching them but the act of

sitting in a dark theater with sticky floors and popcorn-infused, musty anticipation in the air. I'm pretty sure I learned my love of the multiplex from my father. He was severely handicapped in communication too, so it always felt like he took me to the movies instead of talking. And he took me to the movies *a lot*. Maybe he was holding out hope that, in those two hours in the darkness, some made-up words coming out of a made-up person's mouth would resonate with the very not-made-up kid bouncing excitedly next to him. Maybe that would replace all of the conversations we'd never have.

Or maybe I'm just projecting and thinking wishfully. Maybe it was just lazy parenting.

Regardless, I fuck with movies hard. For me, the secret sauce was always that they existed in magical worlds where communication came so easily to everyone. No one was ever truly lost for words. One line always led to the next. Jokes were snappy and perfectly timed, motivations always clear by the end. And stories never lingered. Every action had its purpose, and these tales of heightened reality moved along faster than the speed of normal-ass Brooklyn life.

So of course, at some point I figured I'd moviefy my own life. Just to make it easier for me, you know? Age nine was the perfect time. Especially when Natalie Augustin emerged as the harbinger of my understanding that girls didn't have cooties. She was incredible: a preternaturally sophisticated fifth grader with cow-spotted wing-tipped glasses, a mouth full of rubber-banded braces, and the latest adventures of the Boxcar Children in her backpack at all times. Plus, she always had a full rainbow's worth of colored gel pens ready to share, which I found bafflingly hot. When she auditioned for the school talent show by singing a highly average rendition of Tevin Campbell's "Can We Talk," I was officially hooked. Yes, Natalie. Yes, we *could* talk. And I'd blow her away with the uncanny wit and worldly intelligence she so clearly expected.

We were in the dog days of the fifth grade, just a couple of short spring weeks before graduation, after which we'd all be headed to junior high schools across New York City. One Friday, I sat lulled into a daze by the ne'er deodorized summertime stench of my pre-teen classmates, staring open-mouthed across the classroom at the back of Natalie's head, hoping she'd turn and look at me, when I came to a realization: *my time had come.* I was going to go home that night, pick up the phone, and call the girl of my dreams to tell her how awesome I thought she was. What was the worst that could happen? She'd laugh at my heartfelt honesty, hang up, tell her friends about it, they'd laugh, say I was corny/lame/pathetic, and I'd endure their giggly consternation for the final seven days of school? Fuck it. I wasn't a kid anymore. I was a *young man.* I could take it. I officially had nothing to lose.

But first I needed to prepare. In depth. I was so scared that I'd say the wrong thing / run out of things to say / stumble and sputter my way through my words that I figured I'd script the entire call ahead of time. Armed with index cards and colored pencils, I mapped out every conversational possibility. A choose-your-own-adventure flowchart for the ages. It looked something like this:

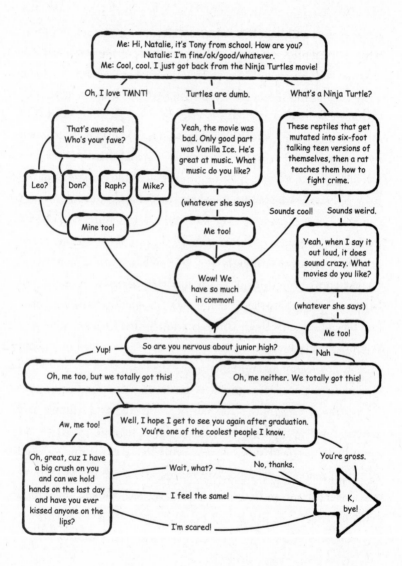

I'm totally not a control freak. I just have the non-stage equivalent of stage fright. Spontaneous high-stakes wording always gave me pit sweats and bubble guts, so I tried to mitigate them with intense scripted preparation. It wasn't that I was trying to control the situation and everyone in it. It was more that I wanted to steer conversations in a direction I could anticipate so that I didn't poop my pants.

Maybe that's just two ways of saying the same thing.

I've always been good at rationalizing my red flags.

I hyped myself up with some pantomimed jump shots and crossover dribbles in my bedroom, brushed my teeth (because you can never be too careful where breath is concerned), picked up the phone, and dialed Natalie's number on that Friday night. Her mom answered and told me that Natalie *wasn't even home*. Why, Natalie? *Why?* I mean, fucking *come on*! How was that the one possibility I hadn't planned for? *Stupid.* Stupid and unprepared. I stuttered my name and call-back number and buried my head under mounds of pillows in defeat.

The next afternoon, Natalie called me back.

And I'd misplaced my index cards.

The conversation went just about as badly as you can imagine. Between unhinged riffing on Ninja Turtle lore, an ill-advised conversational detour into the war in the Persian Gulf ("I'd hate to get killed fighting in the desert. Getting shot and being thirsty sounds super hard"), and laughing so desperately hard at one of her jokes that I squirted some pre-poop into my shorts, I barely got off that call with a shred of dignity intact. Needless to say, Natalie and I never began our grand love story.

Next time I needed a script—and there would be many next

times—I'd memorize my lines in advance. I just had to hope that nobody ever got wise to my handicap.

All of this is to say that art taught me how to (somewhat coherently) speak. And the person I spoke to most was me. I'm not sure if my creativity helped me to understand much about myself. Maybe it could have if I'd paid closer attention. What I did recognize, however, was that my creations let me build out a story: the origins of a character I wished so badly to be. Someone who could navigate life's pitfalls with self-assurance, who could accept the most complex emotions, feel them, grow from them, and move on; someone who always knew what to say and how to say it.

In my mind I built a Tony I could be proud of. Even if he wasn't real, I thought he was the best. Perfect. With a little effort, I could be just like him.

Anything to escape who I actually saw in the mirror. Even as a kid, the mirror only ever left me disgusted. And always disappointed.

The problem is, somewhere along the way I stopped making things. The ideas and images and sounds used to flow through me seemingly of their own volition. I barely even thought about it. But that's the problem with barely thinking about something: you'll never be able to pinpoint the moment when it disappears.

So now it's just me. Me and this formless, seething noise between my ears that I can't turn into anything worthwhile no matter how hard I try. I thought going to the movies would help get my shit back online, just like in the old days, but all it managed to do was let me get super drunk and cry in the dark. No insight. No inspiration. Just red eyes from drunk tears as fake lives unfolded on a big screen.

This shade of life is not enough. It hasn't been enough for a long time.

I think I need a way out.

And I'm a little scared that I don't fully know what that means.

So here I sit. Sweating into a cheaply upholstered sofa as I surrender to Georgia's predawn humidity. Desperate. Smart enough to know that I'm not okay but unable to outsmart myself into fixing anything. In a half-assed attempt to spark some kind of progress, I spent the last hour trying my hand at some amateur photography. If I couldn't draw or compose or dance or sing my way back into sanity's good graces, I might as well see if taking pictures got me any closer. It always seemed like the easiest of the arts—just point and shoot at something that had already done the work of becoming meaningful. Hope the image could pull something silent out of me.

So, of course, the first picture I took was of an old sketch: a candid pencil portrait of me that a friend in college had drawn while I was doing homework. A fucking picture of a picture of someone else's impression of me. That's either a psychological breakthrough or confirmation that my little journey into self-understanding is going to be a complete shit show.

Maybe I'll keep up with the pics. They might end up speaking to me one of these days.

But for now, I've got nothing left.

Except for words.

If I somehow manage to find them and say them aloud or, worse yet, *write them down* . . . fuck. I'm going to be left with no place to hide.

Don't worry. You always find a way to hide.

The fuck?

Oh, shit! You heard that?

Yes, I fucking heard th— Hang on. I know your voice. Damn, it's been—

Years. Yeah. A really, really long time.

Wow. Your voice is deeper than I remember.

Well, I should hope so, since yours is too.

Yeah, that makes sense. So, holy shit! Where've you been? Talking to myself hasn't been quite the same since my good shoulder angel disappeared. Super one-sided.

Where've I been? Dude, you gave me the boot ages ago.

You sure that was me? Sounds like an asshole move.

Given how well I know you, I've operated under the assumption that you got rid of me because I have a tendency to ask you uncomfortable questions in hopes that you'll do better. And you have a tendency to get annoyed by too many of them.

Come on, man. I don't think I'm so fucked up that I'd lock you away just because you're curious.

There's a lot going on beneath the surface layer of your brain, friend. Powerful forces at work.

Okay, let's go on a rapid-fire journey, shall we? It's been a super long time, and I need to gauge how much work we have ahead of us. And how much you've grown, if at all. First question: Why didn't you ever stand up to those white people?

Which time?

Oh, I don't know, how about the time they almost had you arrested for playing tennis with your friends? Or those years in private school when they loved to show you off as long as you kept smiling? Or when they tried to pay you to teach them how to "dance Black"? Or when you joined the workforce and they baited you every day, hoping you'd snap and give them an excuse for getting rid of you? Literally <u>any</u> of those times.

What would have been the point? You know, just as I do, that every year, every new grade, new school, new job, my Black ass was squeezed into their ever-shrinking minority quotas. I've been outnumbered while they held the keys to my advancement and made the rules of engagement. What do you suggest I do when they inevitably act ridiculous, racist, careless, or dumb as fuck? I can't see any option other than just . . . swallowing it. Because I've got to survive. Gearing up for a fight every goddamn day would require energy reserves I just don't have. And honestly, they're not that bad. I've been in their house for so long, their bullshit is just the ugly wallpaper. Might as well get used to it, since it'll always be there, you know? It's the only way they'll let me win.

Only way they'll let you, huh? So tell me, you feel like you're winning right now?

Based on the way you asked the question, I'm guessing I don't.

Fascinating. Feel free to think about it while I switch gears. I been waiting to ask you this one for years: What the hell is it with you and these ladies?

Um, the opportunities are plentiful because I'm cute and my personality rocks?

Do better, ass. You know damn well your longest-lasting relationship was what, eight months?

Probably less.

And would you have even called her your girlfriend?

I mean, we never did the label thing, but I guess we were . . . semiexclusive?

You've been concocting ways to dance around commitment since you were a teenager.

Look, it just never felt right, okay? There's never been a perfect fit, so why waste the time?

"Perfect." That's an interesting goal. Assuming that "perfect" exists, how can you find it when you have so much to hide? You think anyone can fit perfectly between your secrets?

You're definitely overthinking this. Plus, I'm in my twenties. Why should commitment even be the goal right now? I'm a young man and keeping myself open to . . . colorful experiences.

Oh, God, are we talking about the cougar right now?

I mean, we can. Because she was awesome.

Okay, I'm all about having fun. Ask around, I'm a fun guy. But did you feel like you were pushing the boundaries a bit when you said yes to that old lady—

Not old. Old*er.*

Fine: said yes to that "mature" lady who'd been eyeing you from across the bar, and the only words she said to you were directions to her hotel room?

I remember it as a *slightly* more engaging courtship.

Well, particulars aside, you showed up to her suite, where she opened a drawer full of every recreational drug under the sun, and you two ended up getting blitzed off an ambitious combination of weed, ecstasy, and coke. I've been in med school classes with you—that cocaine shit can give you a heart attack, like, real fuckin' quick.

First of all, where's your sense of adventure? Second of all, let's not forget that en route to the hotel I learned that she was a fucking *doctor.* I just had to trust that she knew enough about what she was doing that I wouldn't die there that night.

Okay, drugs and sex aside, wasn't the whole thing a little weirdly . . . premeditated on her end? Like, this grown white lady plucked you out of a club, drugged you to high heaven, and you did anything she wanted you to. There's a one hundred percent chance that she was just fetishizing you. Knocking "sex with a young Black guy" off her bucket list.

So what you're saying is, you're antifun?

You know what I mean.

And to that I say, "Who cares?" We both walked away with a story to tell. I can't be responsible for her cravings for chocolate fondue.

You're so fucking gross.

Dude, you asked.

Jesus, we've got a ways to go. Let's switch gears one last time. Do you have any idea what's keeping you grounded?

I don't think I understand the question.

When's the last time you prayed? What do you pray for? Who do you pray to? Do you even know?

To answer all of your questions at once . . . I don't.

Have you ever considered that placing your faith in something, anything, might make you feel like you have less weight on your shoulders?

Honestly, it feels like pretending that all of my issues aren't on my own shoulders is like playing make-believe. That's why I stopped going to church. Too much make-believe, not enough responsibility.

I get it. You know a whole lot about what you don't believe. Any idea about what you do?

You know, you were definitely right: your ass loves to ask questions. But now it's my turn. Why did you come back?

I think the better question is: Why did you let me out? If I had to guess, I'd say it's because somewhere deep down, you're finally recognizing that your perpetual insistence on traveling the path of least resistance through your life is . . . untenable?

Or maybe I'm just tired and I've lost the energy to keep up any defenses I might have had.

Look, you're right about one thing: you're totally a pain in the ass.

Not sure I ever said <u>that</u>.

But talking to you definitely beats conversations with the other voices I hear in my head. They get a real kick out of watching me fuck up.

Shit. The more I say, the more I worry that I'm losing my marbles. But this is okay, right? Lots of people talk to themselves and don't end up in the nuthouse. I'm just . . . a variant of normal?

Does it matter?

Yeah, I guess it doesn't. Lunatic or not, I'm here. Along with anyone in my head who wants to talk. Great.

Okay. Words. They're my only choice if I'm going to find . . . whatever it is I need to find before I take a tumble off a cliff. Figuratively, of course. Yeah, totally figuratively.

So I'll write. Even though it's infuriating. Even if it takes half an hour to get down even the simplest sentence. Even if my stories aren't worth shit.

Because maybe I'll get lucky and find freedom in these pages before I'm done. Whatever that ends up meaning.

I think that's a good start. I promise I'll take a back seat and keep the annoyance to a minimum. I just want to help you stay honest. Because you lie. A lot. Especially to yourself.

I won't argue with you there.

Plus, you might get lucky and rediscover the muses you lost. They're not as far away as you think.

I'll be on the lookout. If they manage to creep their way in, I'll know I'm on the right track.

So where do I start?
Why don't you tell me the story of Atlanta?

People are funny.

I used to think that when people would ask me every five minutes, "So why do you want to be a doctor?" it was because they were legitimately interested in hearing encouraging tales of my altruism, my academic achievements, and my general menschy nature. Not so. The question is so loaded with preconceived bullshit and poorly veiled agenda that my answer never actually mattered. Older medical gatekeepers—med school admissions officers, college premed advisers, even my fucking childhood pediatrician—would ask it as a prelude to their own lame soliloquies about why I shouldn't pursue doctoring, how hard it would be for me to make the cut, and how I ultimately might not succeed even if I was allowed into the club. Family and friends asked the question to gauge how bonkers I was for sinking so many more years of my life into school, whether I approached freak levels of loving the sight of blood, and how soon they could start asking me questions about their aching back / eyeball / butt cheek.

If I'm honest, now that I'm a few years into the journey, I don't think I have a real answer to the question. I know what I *used* to say: *This is the most noble profession in the world; I just want to help people; I know that not everyone has the capacity to join this profession, so if I do, I feel called to give myself over to it.* Truth is, I don't think I've ever been *called* to do shit. I probably just felt funneled into this path because of my West Indian family. If you're a super smart kid, a bunch of upwardly mobile Jamaicans and Trinidadians will encourage you to be either a doctor (like my

Ph.D. mom) or a lawyer (like my currently disbarred father). These professions are sure things: low-risk, because the world will always be in need of your services, and lucrative, because the world respects your skill set and compensates you accordingly. My family always kept their expectations simple and practical. They never exposed me to or taught me about entrepreneurship or even investment banking—no guarantees in those career paths. I've actually found it fascinating now that I'm an adult: after taking the biggest risk of their lives in moving to another country, my immigrant family became intensely risk-averse in the new world and lives they created.

So why did I want to do this job? Maybe I passively soaked up all of that sweet intergenerational trauma and believed that the best way forward was a low-risk, high-reward, clearly prescribed march to a job everyone would be impressed by. Or maybe I'm just a crazy asshole. (There are actually so many of those in medicine that it would be disingenuous of me to believe I'm the lone normal one attracted to this profession.)

Regardless, I'm here. So what next? Context? That's the backbone of every great tale of the written word, right? Guess I'll give it a shot.

Having recently graduated from Harvard (the fucking epitome of my immigrant elders' American dream), I attended med school in Atlanta, Georgia. At the time that I moved south, I'd never lived outside the Northeast and was still under the impression that New York City was the undisputed capital of planet Earth. If you had no access to late-night pizza, your subway system was made up of fewer than twenty-four interconnected train lines, or your bagels were imported from out of state, I wasn't trying to hear about the "legitimacy" of your city.

Oh, but Atlanta. My dear, sweet Atlanta. A city where every soda is known as "Coke," regardless of name, flavor, or caffeine status. A magical place where total strangers smiling and saying hello to each other on the street was not just commonplace but expected. A spirited town in which everyone was always *finna* go somewhere, or *finna* do something of vital importance.[1] And finally, a land where *it's* can be a conjunction for *it is* or *there is* / *there are* and can be used both ways in the same sentence, demanding that you stay on your toes. (Southern folk, you didn't think anyone noticed that, did you? I've been studying your weirdness. You're on notice.) For example, see this transcript of an actual conversation overheard down south:

SOUTHERN DUDE 1

Pretty cold outside today, huh?

SOUTHERN DUDE 2

Who you tellin'? *It's* so many degrees below freezing that *it's* plenny frozen precipitation in these streets, fam! I'm finna be on my Kristi Yamaguchi on my way to the office!

SOUTHERN DUDE 1

Oh damn. Fantastic contextual reference, bruh!

SOUTHERN DUDE 2

Yahreadyknowwhadideah, bruh.

---

1. *Finna* (pronounced "fnuh"): southern shorthand for *fixing to,* which is southern samehand for *going to.*

Just kidding. Atlantans don't leave their houses during snow flurries. They stay home from work and gaze out of their windows with wide-eyed fear and confusion.

Atlanta provided a colorful backdrop for my medical education, but it was within my school's very expensive and very shiny marble walls that the magic took place. And by "magic" I mean the jarring realization that by making the decision to pursue a career helping my fellow man through compassionate science, I'd entered into a contract with the rest of society not only to learn but also to hold myself to a higher moral, ethical, and behavioral standard than pretty much everyone I'd ever known.

Imagine putting together 120 super intelligent, largely socially awkward kids right out of college and telling them, "Hey, I know you're all still teenagers developmentally, but I'm going to need you to understand immediately that everyone in the 'real world' now looks up to you because you chose to give us your tuition instead of the law school down the street. So . . . act accordingly." That's totally going to go over well, right?

I was slightly older than most of my classmates due to my two-year postcollege life detour. It actually worked in my favor, as the med school admissions committee found my year of teaching high school science, the mysterious circumstances surrounding my sudden resignation, and my subsequent part-time employment at an electronics store slinging iPods to be evidence of my "maturity and commitment to diverse, worldly experiences" compared with applicants who applied straight out of college. The truth was, my body was still learning how to grow hair in all of the adult man places, I was popping juicy zits every other morning, and (most important) I didn't know shit about shit.

None of us was grown. To expect us to be anything more than we were—fucking *kids*—was a recipe for irresponsible shenanigans.

To know Sarah is to hear her coming. Her voice is loud, her laugh is booming, her beer is American, and her personality leaps out with all of the energy one would expect from a girl recently liberated from a life of repressive North Dakotan Catholicism. At a house party during the very first week of medical school, I was standing in the kitchen surveying the dining room table and trying to figure out which of fourteen red Solo cups contained the last of my Natty Lite when a barefoot girl in a tank top climbed onto the counter. She smoothed her denim skirt, blew shocks of blond hair away from her flushed, cherubic cheeks, and announced to the partygoers that, to her horror, we were beering inadequately, and that there was more than enough beer left for us to beer far more aggressively.

She then pierced the bottom of her can with a house key, popped the top, and proceeded to shotgun said beverage to thunderous applause from a kitchenful of drunken future doctors. All I could think about in that moment was how much I hoped her feet were clean, since someone had to cook food on that kitchen counter (because I'm totally normal and these are totally normal inebriated thoughts to have). Once she came up for air from the frothing can, we locked glazed-over eyes. And in that moment, Sarah decided that she liked Tony.

And Tony? He liked Sarah back.

Well, he kind of liked her.

Mostly.

In fact, soon thereafter, Sarah and I entered into an arrangement called "Oh, us? We're just hooking up."

You see, when two people are highly attracted to each other but have dissonant levels of interest in a formal relationship, they will avoid the pressures of traditional "dating" and opt for a much looser form of courtship: getting drunk near each other while their friends are around. Those nights quickly devolve into sloppy make-out sessions, which subsequently lead to sloppy adventures on a surprisingly sturdy IKEA bed frame. This will lead to an eventual naked morning discussion initiated by the More Interested (M.I.) party while the Less Interested (L.I.) party is clearly more focused on the location of brunch:

SARAH, THE M.I.

*(fighting pukey apprehension cramps but
fuck it, here goes nothing)*

So, I was thinking that we could, like, maybe go out to dinner this week.

TONY, THE L.I.

(primarily focused on where the bacon be at)

Yeah, that sounds cool. Who should we invite?

M.I.

(now fully nauseated)

Oh. I mean, we could invite everyone, but I was thinking that maybe just the two of us could do something.

<u>L.I.</u>

(fuckkkkkkk, so this is happening right now?)

Ah. So this is happening right now. Prebacon. Okay, so listen. I think you're amazing, but I just got dumped by someone I really thought I had a future with, and I'm trying to get my mind right about that, so I don't think I'm in the best position to jump into something new right now. I definitely still want us to be cool and hang out, but I totally understand if that's not going to work for you.

<u>M.I.</u>

(it's not fine)

Oh, that's totally fine! You're one of my best friends here, and I totally don't want to make anything harder on you with what you're going through. I'm cool if we keep hanging out. Where's brunch?

And that is the birth of the inherently unstable "just hooking up" relationship.

A year and a half into medical school, everyone in my class was given two months of free time to study for *Step 1*, the first of our medical licensing exams—a super fun eight-hour multiple-choice test that covered all of our medical knowledge up to that point. Sarah and I had decided to study together, which meant spending eight to ten hours a day in a silent room breathing each other's air, often cooking and sharing meals together, and staying in each other's beds multiple times a week. At the time, I wondered if I had stumbled into a bizarre common-law marriage. Thing is, I'm pretty sure that in marriages, one usually has breaks and doesn't spend all day and night with one's spouse for fear of going batshit crazy. This was more like one of those study-abroad, total-immersion experiences. Except instead of French, I was learning about hormone negative feedback loops by day and country-ass barn-wedding rituals by night.

Don't get me wrong, it wasn't all bad. For example, did you know that at some barn parties in Fargo, things get so wild that partygoers will take their shoes off, jump into a cattle trough, and jump around in grain to the sounds of Freddie Mercury? It's called a "trough stomp." And it totally exists.

This routine held up reasonably well for about four weeks, until my classmate Bobby decided his fellow students deserved a New Year's Eve party. This was music to the ears of those of us who had been in town studying seven days a week without respite. Personally, my only daily escape came from the forty-two minutes I set aside each evening for a DVD viewing of an episode of *24*, and Kiefer Sutherland's real-time world-saving antics usually left me more anxious about the fate of humanity than I had been prior. It was time to cut loose.

And cut loose we did. All the familiar trappings of a successful party for moderately well-adjusted about-to-be-professional young adults were in place: iPod playlist, tortilla chips, pounds of assorted dips/cheeses/guacamoles, frozen pizzas, cocktails, cheap beers, and maybe two vegetables. We sang along to Nelly, played frat-worthy games (Flip Cup, Beer Pong, Edward Forty-Hands), and lamented the sorry state of our daily routines. When midnight came, we raised glasses, exchanged high fives, and wished one another luck on the upcoming examination of doom. But when I grabbed my coat and looked around to give Sarah a ride home, she was nowhere to be found.

Wait, Sarah was there? I barely remember her at that party.

'Course you don't, friend, because neither did I. My focus was nowhere near Sarah that evening, and that shit quickly proved problematic.

The next morning, Sarah didn't show up to our usual studying room at school, so I texted to see what time she'd be coming around. Two hours later, I got her response: "I'm not."

Goddamn. Two words with a period at the end? Super short sentence + proper punctuation via text could mean only one thing: she was fucking *furious*.

I arranged for us to meet at her place at the end of the day so that we could talk and I could face the music for whatever I'd done wrong.

"You didn't kiss me at midnight," she said.

Huh?

"You didn't kiss me at midnight for New Year's."

"Was I supposed to?"

Wow, dude, literally the worst possible thing you could have said.

Yeah, I know. Not my finest hour. And just wait, I get worse.

"No, I guess not," Sarah said. She would be unable to look me in the eyes for the remainder of the conversation. That was the moment I realized, and started to miss, just how green her irises were. "I went home and cried until I went to sleep. I just felt so stupid. I know what we said about what we were doing, but I guess I kept hoping that there was something more here."

"So not getting kissed at a party means that there's nothing more here?"

Wow, really knocking it out of the park not coming off as a douche, Chin-Quee.

"Is there?" she asked, eyes on her grainy carpet.

And there it was—the question both of us had been too nervous to ask for the last year and a half. Of course we'd grown close over the last several months, but I had never felt the spark that I'd felt with other girlfriends. At several points over the last year, I'd wondered if that was actually okay. Perhaps this was going to be a new type of relationship for me: truly being friends first, and then allowing those feelings to blossom into something more. Or was it a case of becoming codependent with someone who had become intricately woven into every part of my daily routine? If I were truly interested, would I even be having this debate with myself?

These questions plunged me into the mist of a memory.

A kindergarten-age boy seated on a couch next to his bespectacled father. Young Tony looked up at his dad expectantly and absorbed a casual sermon on love and life.

"Just remember." My father's voice pierced through the haze of memory. "Some girls are just for practice."

I pulled myself back to the present. *Holy shit.* Leave it to my father to plant the seeds of the patriarchy in the mind of a six-year-old. And leave it to my asshole adult brain to wonder if he might have a point. Was Sarah nothing more than a batting practice I'd grown accustomed to as I slogged through the high-stakes, insecurity-breeding days of medical school? A stepping stone toward someone better down the line? Was there a danger in letting her get close enough to hear these whispered thoughts from the darkness? Or should I just calm down and date a nice girl?

Were there humans out there who could answer simple questions about their feelings without a soliloquy?

Was there something more?

"No," I said. Period. Hard stop. I stood up and walked out of the apartment.

At that moment, feeling anything short of sure seemed unfair to Sarah. At least, that was what I told myself as I walked away. My mind, however, was anything but resolute. I went back and forth on the decision every few minutes, starting from the moment I stepped through my own apartment door.

I tried to get back to studying the next day, but I was a fucking mess. Everything reminded me of her, because up until the last forty-eight hours, she had been involved in every single moment of my day for weeks. But this was more than simple practicality. In my newfound solitude, I longed for her effortless kindness, her unapologetic ambition, her generosity in sharing the insecurities she could recognize, and perhaps most of all the comfort and strange familiarity of just how intent upon *being loud* she was. She was smart but not brilliant. Big-boned but not overweight. Someone you'd look right past unless she *made you stop and look*. She was always the first to walk barefoot on a kitchen counter, the loudest laugh in the crowd, the one to lean in for the kiss she wanted, never wait for it. Because if she couldn't be heard, she might just cease to be *seen*.

But I saw her. For a few stolen moments each day since we'd met, I had seen her in all of her boisterous, fractured entirety as only a kindred spirit could. My loudness and need for visibility had been baked into me for years: a consummate performer with a huge smile, wit to spare, and charisma for days. I never quite let myself wonder why I chose high-decibel performance over just simply *being* until Sarah matched my volume. And even then, I was too scared to look in the mirror. Better to just let our similarities entice, intoxicate, and infuriate me.

In short: breakups (even when you weren't *technically* together in the first place) really fucking suck. I even considered starting a support group titled "Grown-Ass Men Who Keep It Real—Real Sensitive, Real Soft, and Really Can't Compartmentalize Their Emotions into a Tiny Box and Shove It into the Back of Their Minds So That They Can Be as Robotically Effective as Society Expects Them to Be." Sadly, the name was too long. And so studying, no matter how many hours I committed to it, was a pointless endeavor.

And then I took the test.

The Step 1 test is pretty damn important. When medical students go on to apply to residency programs—advanced training where we learn the fundamentals of our chosen medical specialties—the Step 1 score is the main gauntlet in the consideration process. Since life is totally fair and always makes sense, there are a lot more medical students in this country than residency spots to accommodate them, and some specialties are more competitive than others. So if you're looking at one hundred applicants for ten spots in your program, you need a way to weed out the "less exceptional." What better way to do that than by picking an arbitrary minimum score on a single eight-hour nonclinical exam and telling anyone who scores lower than that minimum to take a hike?

The maximum (and, to date, unattainable) score on the Step 1 exam is 300. In order to pass the exam, one must score at least 180. The year that I took the exam, the national average score was 222. The average score for applicants matching into otolaryngology, the specialty that would eventually tickle my academic fancy, was 240. The average for neurosurgery was 239. Emergency medicine? 222. Internal medicine? 225. The average score for students at my medical school? 230.

My score?

202.

I'm a high achiever. Always have been. And as such, I've gotten it wired into my brain that I don't have to officially fail at something to *feel* like I failed. Back in high school, I used to mentally self-flagellate after bringing home a 90 percent on a math test—in my book, an A− did not reach my personal benchmark of "exceeds expectations." Then came college, where I tried to force myself to wrap less of my self-worth up in my grades, especially since I stopped getting As once I dropped into the pool of geniuses at Harvard.

I chose to continue to medical school, where math and science nerds who have aligned their success in life with their success in the classroom come to do more of the same. For me, what separated the pressure to succeed at this level from the pressure in college was that I was finally approaching the apex of the What Are You Going to Do with Your Life pyramid. Upon gaining admission to medical school, you are close to the top. But in gaining the freedom to choose what *type* of doctor you'd like to be, every grade and every evaluation weighs heavily, as each will either broaden or narrow the options for what you will be able to do for the remainder of your career.

You can imagine that as I opened the email that led me to my score on that test, I felt a much more profound sense of failure than I had on any examination that had come before it. Not only was I ashamed of my place in the medical student pecking order (though I'd never know for sure, because medical students never, ever share their grades with one another unless they are sure that they are safely at the head of the pack), but a vaguely familiar talking rock had settled into the pit of my stomach that said to me, "You will not be able to be what you want to be."

And having that feeling once you are so very close to the tip of that pyramid?

It makes you feel as useless and discarded as a bag of hot trash boiling in the Staten Island summer sun.[2]

So what did I do? Well, nobody wants to hear the story about the guy who was almost a doctor but quit after he got nervous and sad and moved back home to flip burgers behind the bulletproof glass of a Brooklyn White Castle.[3] Fortunately, that was not my path, and the story of the urban burger maverick is yet to be told.

What I did do was fall victim to blind panic for about seventy-two hours, wallow in self-pity for about a week, and then set up meetings with every senior adviser I could find. They were able to seed the idea in my head that I *might* have a chance at several professional options going forward, as long as I did well in my hospital rotations the next year, showed significant improvement on my Step 2 exam,[4] and chose to apply to a *reasonable* specialty. (Read: a specialty in which applicants tended to have lower average Step 1 scores.)

So I did what any reasonable medical student would do: I decided that I wanted to be an unreasonably elite specialized surgeon. Cue the loser music from *The Price Is Right*. That's right, the one with the sad tuba. That was the soundtrack in my head

2. Fun fact: Until fairly recently, the borough of Staten Island is where the city of New York dumped most of its trash. That's why we make fun of Staten Islanders. Unless they're part of the Wu-Tang Clan. We don't laugh at those guys. They're from SI and hard as fuck.
3. Actually, I might, as it sounds equal parts dangerous and delicious.
4. The "Step 2: Clinical Knowledge" exam tests everything you learn during your hospital rotations and makes sure that you are starting to grasp how the science you ostensibly learned earlier on applies to how people get sick and get better. In essence, they want to know whether you're starting to think like a doctor or if you're stuck in the purgatory of thinking like a chump student.

whenever I told anyone that I wanted to be an ear, nose, and throat surgeon.

And so began my descent into the anxiety-fueled madness that would last for the next eighteen months.

Why did I want to be an ENT? This may be sort of a dickish rationale, but after spending so many years in school and putting myself in hundreds of thousands of dollars of debt, I felt like being a badass surgeon was the only way I'd make the journey worthwhile.

Now, don't get me wrong, all physicians are badasses to a certain degree, but we can all agree that there're levels to this shit. If a patient came into the hospital with something acutely life-threatening, I didn't want to be the doctor who called someone else for help. I was going to be the one who answered that fucking call, knife in hand, adrenaline rushing. As for ENT, these people are experts on the throat and airway. They keep you breathing even when circumstances conspire to suffocate you, and for that reason the specialty went straight to the top of my badass surgeon wish list. Plus, I'm not grossed out by snot, phlegm, earwax, or bad breath. So I decided to apply to ENT residency programs. It'd be a total match made in obnoxious, ego-driven heaven.

There are one hundred ENT programs in the United States. Each program accepts between one and five applicants a year and receives, on average, three hundred applications for those spots. For those of you who need help with division, that means there are not enough spots for all of the applicants. Most ENT applicants apply to about twenty programs to give themselves the best chance of scoring interviews and ultimately matching. I was a below-average applicant, and so I applied to sixty programs all over the country in hopes that I'd somehow manage to slip through the cracks and that someone would find me intriguing enough to interview. To do this, I had to take out yet another loan from the bank, because each residency application costs a little over $100. (Can I get a sad tuba for my credit score's insidious march to death? *Tuuubaaaaaaaaa.*)

Then came the weeks and weeks of rejection letters. Each "We regret to inform you . . ." was a beautifully sharpened, safety pin–caliber tuba knife to my spirit. They didn't regret a damn thing. Politeness has never made the sting of rejection any more bearable. Civility is for first dates and aristocratic dinner parties. Stay out of my hunt for employment.

The average ENT applicant ends up interviewing at twelve to fifteen programs and is often invited to interview at more than that. Out of the sixty programs on my list, I was invited to interview at six. One of these programs was my school's own ENT residency program, which was obligated to interview me whether I had an actual chance or not, as it was my home institution. I was also in direct competition with the only other student in my class who had decided to pursue ENT, who had a decidedly more competitive résumé. You might know her. Her name is Sarah. (*Womp womp womp* for the universe and its trash-bag sense of humor.)

The most common questions I was asked on the interview trail were "What happened on Step 1?" and "So, what's your plan in the event that you don't match?" If we whittle away the bullshit, these are thinly veiled ways of saying, "Bro, you're out of your league here." In those days, I sure as hell felt that way. So I opted for honesty: I bombed the test because I had some relationship drama that came up at the worst possible time and got me too distracted to focus. And if I didn't match? They'd better keep my chair warm, because I'd be back next year with an even more accomplished CV and a chip on my shoulder. It's easy to do away with the convention of sucking up to strangers of a higher station when you're pretty sure you have nothing to lose.

My next step after completing interviews was to enter the Match. The Match is a system created to make the residency assignment process as fair as possible. What it gains in fairness, however, it loses in overall applicant sanity by at least three standard deviations (#C-QMath). The Match works as follows:

1. Every applicant puts together a list of the programs at which they interviewed in order of preference and sends it off to a big computer somewhere in the internet ether.

2. Every residency program puts together a list of all of the applicants who interviewed at their program, in order of preference, and sends it off to the same big computer.

3. The big computer does computer things for about a month, takes into account both the applicants' and programs' rank lists, and spits out a match to both parties on a day in March of the fourth year of medical school. When you enter the Match, you sign a contract stating that you *must* go to the program to which you are matched. No switches. No dropouts. If your Match letter assigns you to your nineteenth choice in Juneau, Alaska, you buy your ass a plane ticket and some mittens under pain of legal recourse.

4. The universe laughs heartily at your illusions of control and self-determination and cracks open another Natty Lite.

With each passing day following the moment I decided on my specialty, I got a bit more nervous, more anxious, and more panicked. Remember when I mentioned the not-so-friendly voices that have taken up residence in my head? This was their time to shine:

an audience between my ears and behind my eyes whose voice transformed slowly each day, over the course of weeks and months, from a rumbling murmur to a hearty nineties-era sitcom laugh track to a well-rehearsed gospel choir singing their hit "Tony, You're a Goddamn Impostor, You're Wasted Potential, and White Castle Is Now Hiring." By the time the day came to submit my rank list, the song was all I could hear every minute of every day. It pulled me away from actual conversations and interrupted my ability to read books and study. In the weeks before Match Day, the remix featuring the hit rap group the Tony You're Worthless and Honestly Not That Good-Looking Either All Stars made its way into heavy rotation.

Goddamn. Torture by way of music. Turning one of the few things I need to survive into an exercise in dry waterboarding. I've got to be the most adept person in the world at being an asshole to myself.

The lyrics started off almost sounding like a joke. That is, until I realized that nobody had the same joke told about them over and over unless it was at least partially true. So the chaotic song played on. And I succumbed to it. It played each morning as I slept in later and later, because what did being on time for things really matter anyway? I grooved to it as I ate a little bit less and poured gin a little bit earlier each day. It was the soundtrack as I stepped into more and more parties (I felt less like a freak when everyone around me was screaming over loud music too), got charmingly drunk, and took girls home with no intention of considering, let alone respecting, their feelings. When the music is that loud, it's hard to remember what feelings actually *feel like*.

By the week before Match Day, the song had morphed into a heavy-metal, rage-fueled cacophony. So fucking loud. I stopped sleeping. Every nerve ending in my body popped and sparked constantly, violently, as I awaited a disaster that felt imminent.

I was teetering on the edge of . . . um . . . Shit, this part's hard.

Try.

I don't even know. Something dark and . . .

And hungry.

I made the last-minute decision to fly from Atlanta to visit a friend in Seattle, because learning to snowboard and possibly hitting a tree and snapping my neck suddenly didn't seem all that scary. I scheduled my flight back to span the window in which I was supposed to receive the Match email so that I'd be able to prolong my limbo just a bit longer.

Of course I couldn't wait. I paid twenty-two dollars for inflight wi-fi and opened an email with the actual subject heading "Did I Match?"[5]

And the entire body of the email read: *Congratulations! You have matched.*

Now, I don't do a lot of morning drinking, but I got *hammered* on that flight back to Georgia and ended up making some louder-than-necessary demands for high fives from flight attendants and appropriately nervous passengers.

For the first time in months, the music stopped.

Three days later, at our Match Day ceremony, I opened an envelope and learned that I'd be packing my bags to move to Detroit, Michigan, to begin residency training. Not my first choice, but definitely not my last, and let's be real: I was lucky to be going to any of the programs on my list at all. And, as an unforeseen bonus, Michigan is in the Midwest—at the very least, I might manage to

---

5. These Match staff bitches were really out here prolonging my anxiety to the very last second? What a bunch of douchebags.

attend a trough stomp party before all was said and done. Plus, rent was cheap because the city's economy had been decimated by the auto industry collapse. And it was cold and snowy for most months of the year, and snow was charming as fuck. So I smiled, hooted, hollered, and glad-handed my classmates, curious to know how many of them, like me, had manufactured their joyous-masks muscle twitch by necessity-driven muscle twitch.

Yup. Cognitive dissonance—it's what's for dinner.

I took a look out the building's windows overlooking the school's courtyard and spied Sarah. She was chatting excitedly with some of the ENT residents I'd met over the past year. The program I'd applied to here had chosen her over me, which was . . . totally fine. Our relationship over the last two years had been a mix of icy and awkward. I had a bad habit of reaching out to her when I was lonely, and she had a bad habit of saying yes when she was exhausted, and those nights reliably ended with a mix of sweat and mutual self-loathing. By day, we didn't speak, as the ferocity of our competition for the same job seemed to intensify in the sunlight. Seeing her gleefully gesticulating across the courtyard during the Match celebration, I felt no relief that our chapter had finally closed, no resolution—only a nearly overwhelming desire to have her in my bed once again. Not for the sake of affection or nostalgia but out of a desperate need to *win* our relationship at the expense of her body and her emotions.

I texted her that afternoon with an invitation to hang out, maybe get a celebratory beer, and oh, there was a new song I'd heard that totally reminded me of her, she should totally check it out. Innocuous enough, right? Her response was uncharacteristically tardy, coming in the form of an email five days later, formal in both voice and format:

Tony,

I've been thinking a lot about us—whatever we were—and I thought I owed you honesty.

I learned a lot over the course of our relationship—specifically, who I am, what relationships can and should look like, and, most importantly, how I view my self-worth. With that said, I do not look back on our relationship with nostalgia. What we had was as stable as a hurricane, and I was naive and immature. At this point, it's time that I move on, and that means a friendship with you is something I can't have in my life.

—Sarah

Well, well, wow. Look who suddenly decided that she could grow up. Just in time to take her victory and run, with no regard for the charismatic, unreliable, emotionally constipated dumpster fire of a dude who helped get her there. No nostalgia? And was that an unspoken undercurrent of regret nestled in the space between her words? Who in the actual fuck did she think she was? I was actively disappearing. My voice was growing weaker and softer by the day. She, of all people, should understand the way I was feeling. And to just cut me off? When I have fucking zero things in my life I can control? And after what she did to me? Fucking with my head right before that damn Step 1 test and tanking all of the prospects I dreamed of? What a wretched fucking b—

Stop. Do better. You know goddamn well that you're having a tantrum because <u>she's</u> what you wanted to control. And you never expected her to stand up for herself.

No, fuck you, that's not it. We were friends! How are you going to just throw away someone you supposedly care about?

She may care about you, but you two were never truly friends, were you? Sounds like she just managed to figure it out before you did.

Fine. This isn't me agreeing with you—you can still fuck off. But I'm just going to take a breath and recognize that I need to respect her wishes. Because that's what a *friend* who *cares* about someone should do. She wants to pretend she's not fractured any-more? Be my fucking guest. But I know it doesn't go away that easily. She'll be back. Nobody wants to be left alone with their fractures for long. Other broken people are the best company.

And I'm quickly losing the energy to remain angry and of-fended. Which I totally have a right to be. It's just . . . the murmurs of the audience in my head. Getting a bit louder now. They must have sensed the hole Sarah left and couldn't help themselves. They love to fill a vacancy. And they just take all of the fucking fight out of me.

A month later I walked across the graduation stage, shamefully clutching my medical school diploma to my chest, feeling as though I'd somehow cheated and that I'd be noosed offstage by a dancing clown at any moment. My mother spent the weekend beaming with pride. My father seemed to have the memory capacity of a goldfish and could not for the life of him remember what type of doctor I was planning on being, despite dozens of prickly reminders. Alas, this was on-brand for him—strangely selective in the details he committed to memory. And of course, his absentmindedness re-garding my accomplishment walked in lockstep support with my intrusive, repetitive self-accusation: I was a fraud.

There'd been a mistake. Numbers don't lie. I shouldn't have made it through. I would be found out. It was just a matter of time. Reasonable, then, that my father refused to remember what I wanted to become. The dream was destined to be short-lived.

Uninspired chuckles from the audience watching from behind my eyes.

Thanks for the encouragement, guys.

And that was four years of medical school.

All leading up to today. The sun's finally up, and I've just taped the last box. The movers will be here in an hour and I'll be on the road this afternoon headed north—in search of fresh trauma in a strange city where my luck at convincing the world that I'm awesome may finally run out.

Hell of a day to start writing.

TWO

A-SIDE—SUCCESS*

After I'd been in these midwestern hospital streets for a few weeks, I found myself reflecting on the old adage that the medical world has cheekily leaked to the general public for decades: "Never get sick in July."

Is it a bit hyperbolic? One hundred percent. But after surviving my first hospital July as a paid employee with a prescription pad and access to needles and scalpels, I can say that the advice to avoid this place in the heart of summer is born of legitimate concerns. Every July 1, the newly minted fresh-out-of-med-school doctors, the *interns*, are let loose across the country to serve the unsuspecting public. On June 30, their coats were dingy waist-length visual reminders of their status as ambitious but ultimately useless lapdogs who weren't even allowed to shake a patient's hand without permission. But on July 1, their coats are knee length, crisp and white, with pockets overstuffed with notebooks, extra stethoscopes, pharmacology guides, and of course the terror that they will be found out as incompetent frauds when asked to make even the most basic medical decisions. And that terror? Completely valid. Because we be fuckin' up. And when we're not fuckin' up, we're scared of fuckin' up.

For those first several weeks of residency, I was afraid of damn near everything. *Am I qualified to perform a thorough rectal exam on this patient? Am I taking too much time finishing my paperwork? Do I tell this patient that this is actually the first time I'm seeing their illness outside of a textbook? Did I just get myself locked in the inescapable stairwell for the third time today?*

Terror at all fucking times.

A hospital visit in July during which intern Tony would be even *partially* responsible for a patient's care was a fate I wouldn't wish on my worst junior high school nemesis. Even Nestor Aguilar, the pubescent asshole who used to clown my bright orange socks. You were a dick, but I wouldn't want to watch you suffer under my shaky hands.

Yet somehow I found in myself an atypically optimistic hope that I'd survive. Maybe even get better. Sure, I'd been chased by a swarm of self-loathing thoughts as I drove north from Georgia to Michigan a few weeks ago, but on arriving in Detroit I decided to adjust my perspective. This wasn't like the beginning of med school, where everyone was expected to know how to study and ace every test right out of the gate. The expectation of interns was that we didn't know a *single fucking thing* about being working doctors. Fear and anxiety were part of the intern job description. So I'd settled into a hope that maybe I'd find a community in the anxious twentysomethings who started the journey with me in July. Maybe we'd be able to share the feelings of helplessness and incompetence out loud, have one another's backs and manage to find our way to healthier, emotionally stable, and fulfilling brain function together. Grown-up maturity was just around the corner. I could *feel* it.

I thought that for about three days. And then:

"Listen, there's one thing you guys need to know about residency," a third-year resident named Mario bellowed over the din of a busy Detroit sushi bar. A number of the surgical interns had been invited out to an unofficial orientation during the first week on the job. We gathered around Mario's portly frame, eager to imbibe any sage advice. He gesticulated with a pint glass, punctuating each word: "First thing you must know, without exception, is your on-call alcohol limit." He wiped sweat from his receding hairline with his forearm. "Now, this is a personal decision, and it's going to be different for each of you, but learn it. And learn that shit right the fuck now." He downed the remainder of his beer and slammed the glass down as he scanned each of us intently, extinguishing any notion that he might be joking. "If you can't do your job after two or three beers, then you're in the wrong fucking profession."

Oh, word? So was I to understand that we were all doomed to desiccate under the pressure and scrutiny of medical training, only to ever be rehydrated by Tito's, Jack, and PBR? I understand drinking as a coping mechanism as much as the next reckless millennial, but drinking as a *survival* mechanism? That seemed moderately troubling.

I watched Mario over the rim of my beer mug as I took another sip. He made a show of playfully distracting a nearby friend so that he could swipe her cocktail glass and down the remainder. Then he giggled like Woody Woodpecker, elbowing a neighboring intern into forced conspiratorial laughter. By all accounts, Mario was a great general surgery resident: he was respected by both his bosses and his colleagues. And yet he'd surely done several surgeries with more than a little bit of alcohol in his system because the job, as he had experienced it, had left him no choice. If he had an internal conflict about this situation, he hid it behind the jolliest of masks.

I had managed to become a master at crafting those same masks for myself. The recognition of an equally skilled artisan doused me in foreboding.

All of a sudden, I wasn't so hopeful.

Drunk-ass Mario had suffered; that much was clear. His booming laughter belied years of open battle wounds. How naive was I to believe that I could endure that same pain without some sort of vice-infused anesthetic? Sure, I might be able to make some friends in Michigan. Confide some of the tough stuff. But Mario had friends too. And here he was.

I had a sinking feeling that my residency friendships wouldn't be about lifting ourselves up.

I scanned the eyes and postures and fingers desperately clinging to alcohol around the table. Residents new and old, sitting side by side but each very much alone.

We wouldn't be friends. We'd be lobsters. Thrown into the same pot. Boiling as a family.

Well, damn, that's pretty bleak even for me.

Yeah . . . fuck, sorry I know I'm usually able to keep the gallows humor yuk yuks coming at a breakneck clip but . . . I don't know, something's been off since I touched down here in Detroit. I think it might have something to do with . . . ah, maybe this sounds stupid but . . . music used to live inside my mind, if that makes any sense. For as long as I can remember, even if I hadn't actually listened to the radio or my headphones in the morning, I'd have a dope-ass soundtrack of beats and hooks and dance breaks in constant rotation between my ears all day long. And now, fucking nothing. I mean, granted, the fact that I tend to hear music other people can't is a likely marker of insanity but . . . man, the silence is way more distracting and distressing than the tunes ever were. And I'm pretty sure it's contributing to my current inability to approach these darker moments with the whimsy you've grown to expect from me.

Maybe there's a way you can keep the melodies close, even if you can't hear them. Find a work-around . . .

Yeah . . . yeah, totally. Maybe I can MacGyver this shit and, I don't know, lightly musicalize this doctor life? Fuck all this doom and gloom. If I've got to write this all down, I'll find a way in that at least lets me grasp for the things that bring me a modicum of joy. Perhaps it's through a collection of my greatest, most formative hits from my early years as a surgeon in training?

Fuck it, I'm on board! I don't really care how you tell the stories as long as you commit to uncovering why you—

Let's be clear: I commit to nothing. This whole mode of wordy expression is new to me, remember? At least let me have fun while I do it. Here's the plan: write down the fucked-up things that happen to me first, engage in introspection second. Or third. Or tenth. Maybe.

All right, I'll take what I can get. For now.

Hell, yeah. Without further ado, I present *The Lil' Dactah Mixtape: A-Side—Success*.*

Track 1: INDEPENDENCE DAY

The on-call room was tiny, measuring about eight by seven feet, with most of the space taken up by twin bunk beds and a wooden desk with a computer that connected me to the ever-changing goings-on of the hospital outside the door. There were actually two doors—one that led to the hallway and the insanity of the patient rooms beyond, and one that led to a bathroom that was shared with an adjoining call room. Thus, any time you were on call at the same time as the constipation-afflicted general surgery resident, every one of his trips to the toilet became a team sport. ("Grab the towel rack and try your best not to pop a blood vessel in your eyeball, Jared. We're going to get *through* this!") There were no windows and questionable ventilation, so the room always felt slightly damp. And finally, the body odor, body sweat, and body hair of the last two or three residents who'd slept there were usually present, as the hospital cleaning crew made it to the call rooms perhaps once every four days. The Holiday Inn Express this was not.

But I was not there for late checkout and a continental breakfast. I was there to doctor. I began my medical career as an intern on the plastic surgery service, and it was *not* as glamorous as it sounds. The days were not filled with fancy face-lifts and nose jobs but with grimy skin infections, hands that had been crushed in car doors, and faces that had gone head to head with steering wheels and lost. For the last three days, I'd been shadowing the junior resident[1] on the service and furiously taking notes on how to write postoperative orders, how to check lab values in the morning, what the best way was to wear my pager (*always* clip it to the waist of your scrubs, *never* to one of your white coat pockets, because you can lose your coat; you can lose your pants too, but it's much more difficult), and what tools actually needed to be in my coat. (Surgeons never carry a stethoscope with them, by the way. Ever. Any television show depicting otherwise is lying to your uninformed face.)

---

1. Junior residents usually have only one or two years of training under their belts but have at the very least learned the ins and outs of the hospital's computer systems and stairwells. A good junior resident can usually begin an appropriate workup for a patient, prioritize the tasks that need to be done, and make their interns appear intelligent to others. A good intern is a reflection of a good junior resident.

On July 4, however, I sat in the call room on my own for the first time and wiped a thin film of condensation from the wall with my finger. As the only representative of the plastic surgery service in the hospital from 7:00 a.m. to 7:00 p.m., I'd been instructed to call my senior resident[2] (who was relaxing at home, presumably getting ready to head out to a barbecue) if I had any questions or needed any help.

Were they kidding me? *Of course* I had questions. I'd been feeling so lost since starting work three days prior, on July 1, that I needed help tying my own shoelaces.[3] But here's the thing about asking for help in residency: you're only supposed to do it as a last resort. The majority of your questions *could* be answered if you did a bit of independent research, and if you *did* call your superior, he or she would always want to know that you'd at least attempted to answer the question on your own. Show initiative, but don't be cavalier. Try to be independent, but don't be dangerous. Trying to find that balance on my first day alone was terrifying. So I sat in the call room wiping questionable moisture from my armrest, willing my pager into silence. But no such luck.

At 11:43 a.m., that little black Motorola box of horrors chirped at me for the first time. I might or might not have spontaneously peed a couple of drops before I got it together. No big deal, right? Happens to everybody?

I picked up the phone and dialed the emergency room. The conversation panned out just like a scene from your average nineties-era fish-out-of-water comedy except significantly less funny, as functioning body parts were at stake.

---

2. Senior residents are responsible for crafting and executing care plans for each patient and delegating tasks to the junior residents. A good junior resident and a smoothly run service are reflections of a good senior resident.

3. Why the hell hadn't I invested in Velcro? Add it to the list of intern-year life regrets.

Emergency Room Resident (ER)

This is the ER.

Tony

(still damp in the pants)

Hi, this is Dr. Chin-Quee[4] from plastic surgery returning a page.

ER

Yeah, um, cool. So listen, we've got a forty-year-old gentleman down here who dislocated his right ring finger when he fell off a bike this morning. We've had a couple of residents and attendings[5] try to pop it back in place but no dice, so we wanted to have the hand specialist come and take a look.

Tony

Yeah, it sounds like you should totally do that.

ER

So . . . are you going to come down, or . . . ?

---

4. Residents never refer to themselves as "doctor" to other residents, so that ER resident 100 percent thought I was a joke before I'd even finished my first sentence.
5. The attending physician is the HDIC (Head Doctor In Charge) and is responsible for the final decisions on all care plans, given that he/she has ostensibly gained a wealth of knowledge over several years of experience. Attendings are rarely interested in the minutiae of *how* things get done. They just want things done, correctly and efficiently.

<u>Tony</u>

(*Oh right, that's me! The hand specialist!*)

Oh yeah, absolutely! I'll be down in a few.

I got on the computer and looked up the patient's X-ray, holding my right hand up for reference, as the number of hand X-rays I'd critically evaluated to that point in my life was equal to zero.

Despite my lack of experience, even I could see that his right ring finger looked funny as hell. Suddenly (and thankfully), anatomical vocabulary came flooding back to me from some dusty med school corner of my brain. There was no evidence of fracture in any of the bones of the hand. The fourth metacarpophalangeal joint (the base of the finger) had been dislocated. The finger seemed to be seated dorsal to (behind) the metacarpal bone, which comprised the "palm" portion of the digit.

I had successfully completed step one: determine that the emergency room wasn't lying to me. Awesome. Now for step two: do something.

But wait, *should* I do something? I had never, *ever* fixed a dislocated finger in my life. Maybe it was time to call my senior and ask him to come to the hospital and show me how to do it?

Nah, eff that noise. Was I really going to call my senior for my first consult of all time without even *trying* to fix the problem? And honestly, what was the worst thing that could happen? I could try and fail and the poor biker's finger would continue to dangle in the breeze. He might be in a little bit more pain, but none the worse for wear. No, there would be no call to my senior. That day, I would celebrate my Independence Day.

To that end, I exercised one of the great freedoms my

forefathers had fought, bled, and died for: the internet search. I logged on to YouTube and typed in "how to fix a dislocated finger." Please hold your applause. Ten minutes later, I walked through the doors of the ER with the tails of my white coat billowing behind me. Emboldened by the treasures of the web, my swagger was fully flexed. The hand specialist was on the loose.

I walked into the patient's room and introduced myself as Dr. Chin-Quee from plastic surgery, the title still ringing false as it escaped my lips. The patient looked up, relieved that "the specialist" had finally arrived. I was immediately struck by how tall he was: easily six foot nine, with enormous hands and long, chubby hot-dog fingers. And of course one of those Ball Park franks was jutting out of his hand at an unnatural angle.

"Aright, Doc," he said, reclining in his oversize spandex riding kit. "Do your worst."

I'd been running each step in my mind for the last fifteen minutes: numb him with an injection of lidocaine on each side of the joint, flex his wrist, stabilize the palm bone with my left hand, hyperextend his jacked-up finger with my right hand, then push the bone back toward its correct position until I felt a pop, drop the mic, moonwalk out of the room, and give the Black Man Head Nod[6] to the first of my brethren I passed on the way out.

But in the moment, I very nearly froze and ran away.

What the hell was I doing there other than playing dress-up in doctor's clothing?

There was an expectant patient in pain waiting for my "expertise," and that impostor bullshit held my hands hostage in my pockets when I needed them most.

---

6. If you know, you know. If you don't, the name's pretty self-explanatory. Just know that it's Black folks' business and carries the utmost social capital.

But then, like a beacon in the night, the voice of Hollywood actor Bill Pullman spoke to me from on high: his iconic speech as President Whitmore in *Independence Day*[7] commenced between my ears. I finally understood the feeling those fighter pilots must have had as their president rallied them to fly out into battle against highly intelligent extraterrestrials with every tactical advantage. And it gave me life:

"We *will* not go *quietly into the night*."

I poked the injection into one side of the finger. *THHHHWIP!*

"We *will not vanish without a fight*."

Injection into the other side. *FFFFFWUP!*

"We're *going to live on*."

And pull the finger slowly backward. *SCREEEEEE!*

"We're *going to survive*."

Push the finger back down toward its natural position until . . . *POP!*

"*Today we celebrate* OUR INDEPENDENCE DAY!"

Well, holy shit. I fucking did it.

My enormous patient knew immediately that his finger was back in place and couldn't stop himself from playing a quick song on an imaginary piano. I, on the other hand, had just realized that I'd been holding my breath the entire time and was trying to ease air out of my lungs as inconspicuously as possible. He thanked me and wrapped me up in a glorious embrace that was one part joyous, one part creepy cuddle from an oversize, bony tarantula covered in spandex. Either way, I definitely needed that hug, so I held on

---

7. One of the greatest cinematic achievements in the history of film/life, *Independence Day* was a 1996 movie about Will Smith, Jeff Goldblum, and a bunch of other true patriots fighting to save the world from a July 4 invasion by ill-tempered aliens. I know every single word of this movie, and I will be taking no questions as to why the entirety of its screenplay takes up real estate in my head that arguably should have gone to things like math.

perhaps seven seconds longer than was appropriate before I wished him well.

"Hey, I think he's all fixed, but you might want to get another X-ray just to be sure," I said to the attending. "You can go ahead and wrap his fingers together for a few days. No need to follow up in clinic."

That was me doing my best "Tony is cool, modest, and respectful even though I'm secretly feeling like the MacGyver of fingers and I deserve ice cream and fireworks" impression. I didn't have the heart to tell them that I'd just learned to do that shit on YouTube. Throwing barbs at their pride was not a cool-guy move and was totally unbecoming of the best hand specialist alive.

They thanked me, I left the ER, and I treated myself to a personal pepperoni pizza from Little Caesars—the only twenty-four-hour food option in the hospital, because we love to give our patients and staff easy access to grease, processed cheese, and early diabetes.

Happy Independence Day, ya filthy animals.

Track 2: PUKE TIME

When my family moved into our first house in Brooklyn in the late 1980s, it was in a dubious state of repair. During the next few years, the house revealed itself to be a true fixer-upper: each of our twelve front steps was of a different height (resulting in several bruised shins); the wooden steps leading down to our backyard splintered to pieces due to a combination of shoddy craftsmanship and an infestation of carpenter bees; and we had one large kitchen pot devoted to catching the water that dripped from the living room ceiling every time someone took a shower upstairs.

To me, none of these was as egregious an offense to my sensibilities as our living room carpet: a thick, shaggy abomination of an indefensible shade of forest green. Initially, it had its own weird charm—lounging on the carpet in front of the television was not unlike lying on a freshly mowed lawn. But just like the grassy knolls of the great outdoors, you never could be too sure what was lurking beneath the surface.

One afternoon I was lying on the carpet, head propped on my hands, watching *Tiny Toon Adventures*. A tiny itch arose on the back of my scalp, so I scratched it. Didn't think twice. A few seconds later there was another itch, this time a bit higher on my scalp. Then another at the very top of my head. Strange, but nothing alarming. I probably just needed to wash my hair that night.

I went to scratch my head again, and as I moved my hand back to my face, I saw something thick and brown fall to the carpet. I looked down to find an inch-long crawly creature lying on its back and wings, six spiny legs kicking frantically in the air. I didn't have to be an entomologist to figure this one out—I'd just spent some time as the playground for a fucking *cockroach*.

To that point in my life, I'd only known raw terror in my darkest nightmares. To feel it during the day in front of Buster and Babs Bunny was something new and overwhelming. My eyes went wide, my limbs froze, and I started that silent screaming thing where your face contorts but the only sound that comes out is hot breath with an occasional pathetic squeak. And then that exoskeleton-having bitch righted itself and scurried back in my direction.

Fuck. That. Shit.

I shot up into the air, limbs flailing, and hopped around the room like a bunny on fire until I ultimately made it to the safety of our couch. I tried (and failed) to get my wits about me as the tiny legs of a hundred imaginary cockroaches crawled over every inch of my skin. Who knew how many other terror bugs hid in those carpet strands? My living room was a living, breathing biohazard.

My (completely rational) fear of becoming a cockroach buffet precluded me from lying, sitting, or even standing stationary on that carpet for damn near three months. My formal requests to have it burned went unheeded by my parents, which was surprising given my father's tendency to spontaneously vomit at the sight of unwanted vermin. He really should have had my back. I was left with no choice but to regularly tuck my pants into my socks as an added precaution when I was forced to spend time living in the living room.

Fuck that carpet.

Sounds like that might have been an unfair conclusion to draw about an inanimate object. I mean, the carpet was just out there carpeting. It didn't choose to invite insects into the mix. Maybe you had an—

Overreaction? Of course I did. That's the point I'm trying to make.

So let's talk about fear: a totally common emotion that we all experience. And it's usually directed toward a specific entity or experience. Some folks are scared of snakes, others of clowns. I've even seen people freak out when they caught sight of pickles. You can be afraid of anything. So the solution is simple: know your fear and avoid it as best you can.

Terror, on the other hand, is uncommon. In my experience, it erupts when something you fear appears in a place you don't expect. It's often so powerful that the lasting effect after terror has worn off is a *multiplication* of your fears. For example, let's say you really don't fuck around with snakes—they eat their food whole, and it's totally unnatural that something can move that fast on land without legs. They're clearly God's mistake, right? And totally reasonable grounds for ophidiophobia. So you avoid places like tall grass and that trash *Anaconda* movie starring Jennifer Lopez. It's pretty easy to live a snake-free life.

But what if one day you're out in the countryside, you need to go to the bathroom, and your only option is the outhouse? As you squat down on the outhouse toilet, a snake creeps up underneath you and bites you in one of your cheeks all the way down to the dark meat. You'll freak out, run, scream, and hide in your cabin. The next day, you go home not only more scared of snakes but also scared of outhouses, and possibly afraid of all toilets. You feel me now?

Consider yourself felt.

After the carpet debacle I wasn't just super scared of bugs. To this day, I have an irrationally aggressive stance on floor-bound fabric. Fuck that scary-ass carpet and all of its shag carpet–ass friends.

Three weeks into my first month as an intern, I was finally settling into a routine. It was my last week on the plastic surgery service, and I'd started to find some security in the day-to-day repetition: go see a consultation; gather information; report back to my junior resident, who'd send the report up the food chain; get instructions; follow directions; rinse; repeat. So I thought nothing of it when I received a call from the ER requesting that I evaluate a hand wound.

I pulled the curtain back at the patient's doorway and found a woman in her late sixties looking up at me with a high-wattage smile. Caramel skin with freckles, hair bound by a playfully patterned cloth, she was midgiggle, wrapping up a light moment that I'd just missed. A heavyset woman in a flowered scrub top sat in a chair beside the patient's bed, arms folded, gaze fixed on the linoleum floor. I thought back to the review of the patient's chart I'd done a few minutes earlier, and the relationship became clear: the woman smiling up at me, who appeared otherwise healthy, was named Nora and suffered from severe dementia. She was a resident in an adult care facility, and the woman in the chair next to her was her nurse chaperone. The joke I'd walked in on had probably been told by Nora to an audience that included only herself.

I walked in and extended my hand in introduction. Old Nora reflexively reached to meet me but stopped short, glancing down at her own hand. Her eyebrows furrowed as she slowly remembered why she was in the emergency room: her right hand was wrapped in what appeared to be several feet of cotton gauze fashioned in such a way that it seemed she was wielding a snowball. In the moments that her hand was extended toward me, the stench crept into my nostrils. I remember it distinctly as one part skim milk left out to ferment in the sun, one part dead hamster carcass.

"What happened to your hand?" I asked.

Nora smiled up at me dreamily. "Oh, it's that darn bug bite that just won't go away."

Bug bite. Right. I asked the question once more, this time to her nurse.

"We haven't been able to get her in to see her primary doctor yet, so we've just been wrapping it up," the nurse replied, her eyes still cast down. "The smell just got so bad this week that the other residents started complaining."

Yeah, no shit. And this sweet lady had no idea her hand smelled like a wet dog that had eaten another, very dead wet dog. I knew

I'd find nothing good beneath the bandages. So I recited the sentence that everyone has heard from their doctor at some point in their lives—words meant to betray a certain eager fearlessness but that, as I'd already learned in my three-week career, often represented nothing of the sort: "All right, let's take a look."

To the credit of the nurses at her facility, Nora's hand had been nearly mummified by several feet of gauze, wrapped so tightly it would have made a professional boxer proud. I rolled the ribbons of gauze away until I reached the last bits of dressing, which were stuck in place by murky brown fluid emanating from the wound, at which point I whipped out a pair of scissors from my coat pocket and finished the job.

At first glance, it seemed as if she were simply holding a flesh-colored softball in her hand. On closer inspection, however, I could see that the ball was actually *a part* of her hand. The creases of her palm and the skin on the back of her hand were stretched over a grapefruit-size mass bisected by her fingers, which lay limp and useless around the edges. On the palm side of the ball the skin had eroded, leaving a crater two inches wide. The depth of the crater was unknown, as it was filled with tiny grains of rice.

I'm sorry, what? Had the caretakers at the nursing home tried to quell the stench of her rotting hand with a couple of scoops of Uncle Ben's? I opened my mouth to ask the nurse about the benefits of medicinal grain therapy when my breath caught in my throat. The rice grains were *moving*—purposefully sliding over one another, scurrying in and out of the crater. This wasn't a case of the magical healing rice of fairy-tale lore. I'd read stories about these things but never seen them with my own eyes. These were *maggots*.

The silence surrounding my realization was pierced by the sound of carbonation bubbles from a freshly poured glass of soda.

Again reason crept in—nobody in the room had opened a can of Coke, nor was anyone eating a bowl of freshly milked Rice Krispies. The barely audible snaps, crackles, and pops were coming from the putrid crater in the woman's hand. It was the sound of maggots eating dead flesh.

"How does it look?" Nora's voice wafted softly toward me. "Have you ever seen anything like this before?"

So. *Puke time* is a phrase I coined a few years ago, during my days of excessive recreational alcohol consumption in medical school. It's the amount of time between the start of that sickening hypersalivation in your mouth (known in medical circles as *water brash*) and the moment you actually vomit. Through trial and very messy error, I was able to identify my personal puke time as twenty-two seconds. It was remarkably consistent and long enough to allow me to make a beeline for a bar's restroom after a shot of tequila and, if all stalls and urinals were occupied, still have eight to ten seconds to get out the front door and vomit on the sidewalk like a pro. Flattering? No. But necessary if I was going to keep hope alive that I could still make out with the drunk girl I'd been giving drunken eyes to all night.[8]

Once the maggot situation fully dawned on me, that puke-time water rushed into my mouth. At the same time, my deep-seated carpet-cockroach terror came crashing in, bringing with it the sensation of hundreds of little maggots crawling up and down my skin, bathing me from head to toe. I was paralyzed, my eyes fixed on the horrifying maggot spectacle. And I had approximately eighteen seconds left before I threw the fuck up, so I was doing *great*.

---

8. And just to clear the air: yes, I've puked then made out with a nonzero number of women. I (usually) gummed and rinsed first, but I can concede that it was a pretty gross move.

I was only able to pull myself back from the brink of frozen terror by focusing on three of the simplest thoughts I could manage:

1. Be nice.

2. Get out.

3. Do not vomit on this woman.

The tissue deep inside the hand wound was dead. That's why it
was infested with maggots; they actually eat dead tissue, so in
their own disgusting way, they were keeping the wound fairly
clean. Trying to remove the maggots wouldn't help matters right
now. The best move would be for me to wrap the hand up in gauze
as it had been before, maggots and all. We would come up with a
plan for this later, after I spoke with my senior residents.

Be nice. I forced a smile. "Oh yes, I've seen this plenty of times."
Lies. "Don't worry, we'll take good care of you."

I began briskly rewrapping the wound with fresh gauze, but—
and this is crucial—my puke timer was down to three seconds.
Get out. No longer an option. *Do not vomit on this woman.* God
help me.

It was happening. I'd managed to go around her hand a few
times with the gauze when my stomach gave a couple of preliminary
retches. Then up it came: hot, bilious juice rushed into my mouth,
filling my cheeks as I willed my lips into a watertight seal. I was 100
percent sure that my cheeks were finna burst. I couldn't breathe,
tears clouded my vision, but somehow I had the presence of mind to
bend my head down toward my own shoes. If I was going out as the
great American puking resident, I would *not* vomit on this woman.

I awaited the next wave, the one that would force hot emesis
out of my lips and turn me into the smelliest fountain statue of all

time. But by some act of divine providence, it never came. I saw my chance. Carefully, methodically, I swallowed. Three enormous, burning gulps, sliding my own vomit back into my esophagus. I silently gasped cool air into my lungs and looked up at Nora, my eyes moist with tears. She was smiling just as she had when I first walked in, oblivious to the tragedy that had nearly befallen her. Her nurse hadn't flinched, her eyes on the same cracks in the linoleum floor. I should have puked on her shoes just to see if she was capable of purposeful movement.

I finished wrapping her hand and excused myself, making quickly for the restroom, where I frantically rinsed my mouth, dabbed my bloodshot eyes, and held on to the sink as aftershock shivers of maggot terror shook my body.

Then I went back to work.

Nope, you're not getting off that easily. I know you can dig deep to find an uplifting moral buried somewhere in all of those maggots.

Nope. I hate this story and wrote it only because it was traumatizing as fuck. I mean, maggots, rotting flesh, and puke swallowing? What kind of trash job would force me to experience shit like this, then continue on with my day as if nothing had happened? Plus, the grapefruit-size tumor / maggot residence had rendered the hand unsalvageable, and we ended up having to amputate it. *Plus,* the tumor turned out to be a fucking cancer and now she has to go through God knows how many debilitating treatments in the fog of dementia with a fucking hand stump. Worst. Story. Fucking. Ever.

Okay, now that you've gotten the whining out of your system, you wanna try again?

Fine. For anyone who's considering patient care as a career: at some point, this line of work will put you face-to-face with something that ensnares you in a primal, irrational panic. You will want to run and hide. You will want to cry. You will want to throw up. Just do your best not to, because the people in your care (and the people who write your check) expect you to have evolved past normal human reactions and emotions. Despite the fact that your job carves out new fears and extracts new terrors by the minute, your constant state of posttraumatic stress doesn't fucking matter. It's completely unfair, but the belief that you won't run, cry, laugh, or vomit actually helps people feel a bit more human when they have been treated outside the hospital as anything but. So put on your big-kid pants, exchange your own humanity for someone else's, compartmentalize your unruly emotions, and pack some extra gum—that postvomit swallowing breath can haunt you for hours.

And for any future patients: if a doctor or nurse ends up puking all over you, use whatever energy you have left to take it in stride and forgive them. Trust me, they tried their best.

Track 3: PLUMBING

Here's something I learned fairly early on in my medical career: most surgery is all about fixing the plumbing. Our wondrous human bodies are driven by a masterfully crafted system: pipes for breathing, conduits to deliver blood, tubes for food digestion, and hoses that allow for the culmination of bedroom activities. Should any of your plumbing malfunction, surgeons can be your personal Super Mario Bros. Leaky pipe? We got you. Pipe clogged? We are human Drāno. You got something going down the wrong pipe? We don't stand for it. Oh, the Drāno didn't work? We'll get you a whole new pipe. Might even make it out of some of your other pipes!

My first plumbing emergency sang through my pager on a frigid day in January of my intern year. I was on my ENT rotation, so I was finally under the tutelage of the residents and staff with whom I'd continue to work closely for the next several years. For me, this was the most important rotation of the year, as it served as a two-month-long first impression to my future lifelong colleagues. As a result, the pressure level had gone from "New England Patriots' Super Bowl Deflated Game Ball Low" to "Raw Egg in a Microwave High."

Oh, shit, I remember the egg fiasco! Wasn't that Janet from down the hall back at Harvard?

Good memory! Granted, your memory is mine, but impressive nonetheless. Way back once upon a time, when I had nary a chin nor chest hair to speak of, I was a seventeen-year-old freshman at Harvard University. For all of its mystique and clout, in the end I'm pretty sure Harvard is nothing more than a really expensive, fucked-up social experiment for smart kids. Everyone on the planet knows the name *Harvard*. Lots of people dream of going there, and because the school accepts fewer than 5 percent of its sixty thousand valedictorian applicants each year, everyone assumes that the kids who make the cut are supergeniuses. And that includes the kids who are accepted. No student would ever say it out loud, but each of us assumed that the student sitting next to us was the next Albert Einstein or Stephen Hawking or Barack Obama. And that shit right there was *stress full*, because at the end of the day, we were fucking teenagers. And teenagers do dumb shit. But doing dumb shit around your closeted-genius friends? That was a big no-no. Being exposed as the one nongenius who'd managed to slip through the cracks was a constant source of anxiety for all of us. At least, I hope it was all of us and not just me. I never knew for sure. As I said, we never talked about it. You could meet someone and become the best of friends, but if either of you was suffering academically, you did that shit in silence.

Damn, now that I think about it, it was actually great med school / residency practice.

There were four dudes in my freshman-year dorm room: one serious white guy (math genius and future military tactician / food delivery app founder), one silly white guy (loved to read American history nonfiction for fun, future wunderkind investment banking partner), one first-generation Indian guy who couldn't do his own laundry (future CEO of a nonprofit that would teach governments worldwide how to provide their citizens with clean drinking water), and me, a Black kid from Brooklyn who liked to sing and dance and struggled to keep up with the assigned reading for all of my classes. Together we'd decided that we could become the social hub of the entire dorm with a single purchase: a microwave. Everyone needed one but not everyone had one, so we allowed people to pass through whenever they wanted to heat their food, and we'd provide the stimulating conversation. One day, Janet from down the hall popped in, told us she was going to hard-boil an egg real quick, placed an egg (still in its shell) on a paper plate, set the microwave for two minutes, and then left without the customary small talk—a highly rude breach of decorum.

It was the first time I remember experiencing the absurd power of white women. Janet was super Caucasoid and movie-star hot, and she entered every room and interaction with the confidence that she should be welcome and listened to. And I'd fallen victim. It was completely nuts that she'd walked into my room and told me some wild cooking shit that was clearly outside the realm of possibility, and my first thought was "Damn, Janet must be on the cutting edge of egg boiling."

Damn, these white girls really need to learn to use their powers for good.

You're telling me. Janet chose to defy the basic principle of boiling, and so cruel science took the wheel. After about forty-five seconds, that egg fucking exploded. The door of our little microwave blew clean off its hinges, and hundreds of pieces of partially cooked egg rained down all over the room—on my computer, on the ceiling directly above the microwave (somehow), and on my poor Indian roommate's hair and shirt (no worries, though, his mom was dropping off fresh clothes for him on the weekend).

Janet was super sorry and promised to get us an even better microwave, which she never managed to do.

I had the feeling that no matter how many appliances she cheerfully broke along the way, Janet would end up just fine. And I was right: last I heard, she is responsible for teaching Google how to Google or something.

Damn. White people. Blowing shit up and leaving us to clean up the eggs since the beginning of time.

Tell me about it. Hopefully I can manage to bring this egg analogy full circle.

One January morning, I sat down at a nurse's station to return a page. The report from the resident came quickly: *Your patient in the ICU is having desats, and we're not sure why. Can you come up and evaluate her?*

Desats, or desaturations, are drops in a patient's measured levels of oxygen in the blood. As most people know, oxygen is necessary for continued human life, so if there's not enough of it in the blood being delivered to your various body parts, that's a problem.

And if the reason for the desaturations is unknown, it can be a complete nightmare.

I hung up the phone, grabbed my tackle box,[9] and ran to the patient's room. I dabbed sweat from my face and neck with a white coat sleeve, adjusted my glasses, and took three slow, deep breaths—despite my rookie status on the wards, I'd already learned that having even the *appearance* of panic or disorder could turn a high-stress event into a catastrophe. Plus, I have always had a major sweating problem and my pits had been soaked underneath my coat for at least two hours already. There would be no disrobing during this emergency. No matter how hot the pits are, just look cool. Cool is competent.

I strode into the room and quickly took stock: My patient, a petite woman in her forties, lay motionless on the bed, save the rhythmic, mechanical rise and fall of her chest and belly. She was not breathing on her own—a tube, taped to the left corner of her mouth, connected to another tube that connected to another tube that connected to the ventilation machine (so much redundant plumbing). The respiratory therapist (easily identified by her black scrub top) danced between the machine's monitor and the tubing connected to the patient. She was the one in charge of the vent settings and seemed to be searching her equipment frantically for malfunctions. Her pit sweat level: six out of a possible ten.

I turned my attention to the monitor above the patient's bed,

---

9. ENT residents carry around all sorts of face hole–related tools—tongue blades, snakelike flexible nasal scopes, even inflatable nasal tampons for stopping stubborn nosebleeds. At my hospital, we decided to throw them all into a fishing tackle box for safekeeping. As the junior resident, it was my responsibility to keep the box stocked at all times with everything I or the rest of the team might need. It was also my responsibility not to lose it somewhere in the hospital, which, in those early days, would happen to me three or four times a day.

where her vital signs were displayed in a variety of neon colors, and registered them all in a matter of seconds: Blood pressure 118/70. *Good. Within normal limits.* Heart rate 128. *A little too fast. Her body is just starting to panic.* Oxygen saturation 90 percent. *Okay, but not great.* A normal human with normal lungs should be able to sat greater than 95 percent if all is well. For some reason they were not able to get her up to that level, even with the help of the ventilator. I continued to scan the room.

A nurse stood at the bedside computer in a brightly flowered scrub top, calmly entering notes into the system, preparing to administer a medication into the patient's IV line. Pit sweat level: two of ten. This was not her first rodeo. My eyes turned, finally, to the ICU resident standing at the foot of the bed, arms folded, brow furrowed as he stared intently at the vital signs. I'd done the same thing several times over the last few months. Out of ideas, he was attempting to right the patient's vital signs through sheer force of will. Sweat bubbled on his forehead and dripped down to the lapel of a crisp white coat, still creased from its earlier life inside vacuum sealed plastic. Pit sweat level: nine, without a doubt. He was an intern. Just like me. And he was freaking out.

He caught my eye. I introduced myself. He spoke.

"Oh, man, thanks so much for coming so quickly. So this lady was doing just fine until about fifteen minutes ago, when she started to desat. We've been able to keep her oxygen levels up by increasing the pressure on the vent, but even with that she's just hovering around ninety percent."

The story seemed to be missing a bit of key information. This lady was not super sick otherwise, and her lungs had been working well enough as of that morning. By "increasing the pressure" he meant that in order to keep her oxygen up, he and the nurses had set the ventilator to start blowing air into her breathing tube harder and faster. Not a great permanent solution, as high pressure for too long could cause legitimate damage to her lungs. There had to be a plumbing problem that was being overlooked.

"Did anything happen fifteen minutes ago that might have de-stabilized her?" I asked. "Was she rolled around in her bed? Did someone sit her up or down quickly?"

The intern shrugged helplessly. He had no idea, and I had the feeling that he hadn't asked.

A meek voice from the corner said, "I adjusted her breathing tube." I looked over to the respiratory therapist, who had finally stopped tinkering with her machinery. "When I came into the room, I saw that the tape on her endotracheal tube had come loose, so I retaped it to the side of her mouth."

"And then we started having problems?" I asked.

She nodded. Jackpot. Now we were getting somewhere.

The reason that this patient was in the hospital was because she had a rare condition called a *tracheoesophageal fistula*. It's a mouthful, I know. And can be a pretty deadly mouthful at that. Let me break it down.

The trachea, also known as your breathing tube, starts in the middle of the neck and extends down into the upper chest, where it splits in two—one path leading to the left lung and one to the right lung. The trachea is big, wide, and firm—it doesn't stretch much and is hard to break, like an oversize sipping straw.

The esophagus, also known as your swallowing tube, also starts in the middle of the neck and extends down into the upper chest, where it empties into the stomach. The esophagus is also big, but its walls are soft—it needs to stretch and move chunks of food and drink down toward the stomach. In the spirit of keeping our analogies consistent, let's say the esophagus is more like an oversize sour straw candy, only it's 95 percent less delicious.

Not only do these tubes both start in the neck, but they are also stuck together like conjoined twins: the trachea sits in front (you can feel it in your neck if you try—it's the firm, ridged tube in the middle of the bottom part of your neck, and if you push on it hard enough you can make yourself cough), and the esophagus sits right behind it (sorry, you can't feel this one by poking yourself in the neck). The back of the trachea is tightly connected to the front of the esophagus. The oversize sipping straw and sour straw are essentially glued to each other as they travel down the neck to their respective destinations.

A fistula is just a fancy medical word for an unwanted connection between two systems in the body. In this patient, there was a very unwanted hole between the back of the breathing tube and the front of the swallowing tube. So air could get into the esophagus from the trachea (not the biggest of deals, save the unsavory belching that might result). More important, food and saliva could get into the trachea from the esophagus. This in turn could lead to food and saliva in the lungs, and that is *not* a good thing for your quest for continued life on planet Earth.

This patient had been brought into the hospital because she'd developed a pneumonia (or lung infection) as a result of too much food and saliva getting into her lungs. She'd become too weak to breathe on her own, and so a breathing tube had been placed in her trachea so that the ventilator could do the breathing for her. She'd been steadily improving for three days, until fifteen minutes ago, when her breathing tube had been adjusted.

I shut my eyes to try to visualize the problem. She'd been doing fine. Breathing tube was moved. Then she started doing worse. She was still getting oxygen, but not enough. The only way to get enough air to her lungs was to increase the rate and pressure of the air entering the tube. And it seemed to be working: her chest and belly were rising rhythmically.

Wait. Her chest *and* belly were rising? That couldn't be right. I approached the bedside for a closer look. Her chest rose up and down with each breath, as it should. Her belly seemed to be rising and falling as well, but on closer inspection it was just getting bigger. A fat belly on a lady who had been skinny last night. I placed my right hand on her belly and pushed gently. The top of her abdomen felt like a fully inflated balloon.

We weren't just ventilating her lungs. We were ventilating her *stomach.* All because of the hole between the straws.

Well, shit. This was a problem.

I whipped out my phone, excused myself to the hallway, and called my chief resident. This wasn't the time for YouTube-supplemented pride. Even with only a few months of training, I knew that if I got this wrong, this lady was going to die due to lack of oxygen.

Kenny picked up on the fourth ring, and I launched into the story. When I'd finished, there was silence on the other end.

"Okay," he began, "I think you're definitely right about her tube being in the wrong place, and it's likely above her fistula. We're going to have to plan on taking her to the operating room to secure her airway today. But right now, she's unstable. I'm about twenty-five minutes away, but I doubt she'll last that long. I need you to put her breathing tube back in the right place."

Oh, right. Just pop it back in the right place and save her life before her lungs suffocate and her belly explodes. No big deal.

Kenny could sense the apprehension in my silence. "Just grab a scope, disconnect her from the vent, put the scope down her ET tube, figure out where the hole is, and guide the tube past it. I'm getting in the car right now, so I'll be there as soon as I can."

(*Click.*)

All right, then. There'd be no further questions, I guess. I turned my eyes back to the patient's room, where all three staff members were looking my way expectantly. I strode back into the room and broke down the plan for them: "The breathing tube is likely in the wrong place and is pumping air into both the lungs and the stomach through the fistula. I'm going to slip a foot-long flexible camera down the tube and guide it back into the right place."

The team nodded, and I opened my tackle box. I could *totally* do this. I'd scoped dozens of people up to that point. Perhaps not exactly like this or under this sort of imminent-death time crunch, but I could think my way through. Just relax, breathe, and, of course, find the flexible scope.

I'd been rummaging through the contents of the box for several seconds and had found nothing. Where was the scope that I'd brought with me? Rule number one of being an ENT junior resident was to always have a scope in the box at the ready. And I always had.

Except for the last twenty minutes, because I'd left it upstairs in the ENT clinic to wash and disinfect.

Fuck. Me.

The consult I'd just come from hadn't required the flexible nasal camera, and I'd been on my way back up to grab it when the call for my ICU patient had come through. I looked up at her vital signs just as the oxygen saturation ticked from 90 percent to 89 percent. When someone is losing oxygen, their body can usually hold their sats at or above about 90 percent for quite some time. But once they drop to 87 or 88 percent, the oxygen in their blood can plummet within seconds.

She was running out of time. And I was the jackass who had left the one tool he needed on the other side of the hospital.

I turned to the sweaty intern. "I've got to run up to the clinic to grab a scope for her. I'll be back in two minutes."

I caught the quickest glimpse of his expression—confusion laced with just a dash of helplessness—before I walked briskly out of the room and into the hallway. Honestly, it was probably going to take closer to five minutes to get to clinic and back, but I didn't want the neck-sweating intern to panic just yet. I pushed through the ICU's double-door exit. And then I ran.

Start the motherfucking microwave-hard-boiled-no-water-egg timer. Except this time the egg was both my brain and some poor lady's life.

Dansko is a shoe manufacturer that makes a very distinctive model of "professional clogs." They are made of firm leather, lift you to a full inch taller than your natural height, slip on and off your feet quickly, and are unbelievably durable. Perfect for a profession full of people with Napoleon complexes who don't have the disposable income for yearly trips to Payless. However, despite all of their virtues, cross-trainers they were not. As I took off through the wards, I reminded myself that footwork would be the limiting factor: *Your traction is low, so slow down on those corners and don't take them too tight. You've got no kind of ankle support to speak of, so WATCH THAT LATERAL MOVEMENT, YOUNG CHIN-QUEE!*

I sprinted past staircase number 1—those stairs went only as far as the sixth floor, and I needed to get up to the eighth. Bolting through the wards, patient rooms blurring past on either side, I wove between groups of chatting nurses and loitering med students at top speed. As the way cleared before me, I was feeling strong. Athletic, even. Then, as if on cue, a rolling bed rounded a corner up ahead and, propelled by an acne-ridden volunteer, cruised toward me, initiating the most unfortunate game of chicken in the history of metro Detroit. As I barreled toward this certain head-on collision, I saw only two options, and they were both awesome:

Badass option #1: Pick up some speed and at the last moment jump as high as I could, complete a full flip in the air, tuck my legs so that I'd narrowly miss the ceiling and land Spider-Man style on the other side of the bed, stand up in slow motion, give a nod to the pubescent volunteer, and then be on my way.

Badass option #2: Line up the angles just right, run *Matrix* style up along the wall of the hallway, get about two full strides along the wall before gravity nudged me back to Earth, stick the landing, grab the closest pretty lady, consensually kiss her on the mouth, and then break back out into my sprint.

It was time for a hero. I went with option two. Once I was within five feet of the stretcher, I juked to the left and immediately felt searing pain bloom in my right ankle. Instead of taking a great, gravity-defying stride up the tile wall, I crashed shoulder first into a wall-mounted metal chart locker and crumpled to the linoleum floor. My ankle was definitely sprained. I'd gotten too cocky, and my Danskos had brought me back down to Earth.

I straightened my glasses, looked up, and saw a pretty lady in circus-print scrubs standing over me, her face caught between concern and stifled laughter. "My God, are you okay?" She offered me her hand. "That looked pretty bad."

I dug through the pain in search a super cool thing I could say to save face, but all I managed was a croaking "Nunnnghhhhhhh." Smooth, I know. I shamefully took hold of her hand, pulled myself to my feet, turned, and broke back out into a sprint, each step punctuated by pain that shot out of my right ankle like lightning.

I passed another staircase at the end of the ward—this one did go up to the eighth floor, but I'd learned earlier that year that all of the doors were locked from the stairs side. If I hopped in there, I'd be trapped until some Good Samaritan let me out. What kind of sick bastard designed this fun house?

I gingerly rounded the next corner, blazed past a set of elevators, and dived into the next staircase on the right. I emerged on the eighth floor after taking the steps two at a time, bounded through the door of the ENT clinic, and made a beeline for the scope washroom. I snatched the scope from its bath of cleaning solution, rinsed the tip in the sink, dried it with gauze, attached a battery pack, and turned back to the clinic door. I could hear my heartbeat in my ears, and each breath burned in my chest. My patient was four floors down and slowly suffocating. Just one more sprint.

The entire way back was clear of obstructions, and I arrived at the door of my patient's room in the ICU in two minutes. I paused once again, wiped my brow, and attempted to slow my breathing. Time to work.

I strode into the room, doing my best to mask my limp. The air was noticeably tenser than when I'd left. I took in the vital signs: Blood pressure 90/70. *Too low. Not good.* Heart rate 156. *Way too fast for someone not out running a marathon.* Oxygen saturation

72 percent. *Way too low. She didn't have enough oxygen to sustain normal body functions, so she was not just panicking—her body was starting to go into shock, also known as emergency mode. And shock didn't last for long.*

The sweaty resident spoke quickly to the nurse as she drew drugs up into small syringes. The respiratory therapist was no longer alone, muttering rapidly to her newly arrived supervisor, hands on the endotracheal tube, which was no longer taped to the patient's face. *No. They've been moving it. Why didn't I tell them not to move it?*

"Hey, everyone, I'm back!" My voice sounded as if it belonged to someone else, because clearly there was *no* way that I was qualified to be in charge of this emergency. Nonetheless, the words kept coming. "So here's the plan: When we're all ready, you folks from respiratory are going to disconnect your machine from the endotracheal tube. Then I'm going to slide my scope down the tube and see where we are. I'll reposition the tube, and as soon as I take the scope out, I'll be the one to reattach the ventilator. I'll hold it in place while you start the machine and breathe for her. Does that sound good?"

Nods of assent all around. Her oxygen saturation ticked down to 70 percent. In the sea of bleeps, blips, and screeching alarms that sound when a patient in a hospital is in distress, there was one alert that my ear had already learned to hear through them all: every two seconds, there was a short, high-pitched beep that informed me of her level of oxygen saturation. Every time the oxygen level dropped, the pitch dropped just slightly, as if someone were having trouble playing a very sad and monotonous piano scale. I wouldn't be able to see the oxygen levels while I was looking down the breathing tube, but I would be responsible for knowing them.

I would have to listen for the music of one set of beeps in a sea of emergency alerts.

Sixty-nine percent.

Go time. Scope in hand, I approached the patient's bedside. My head felt overinflated and poised to pop. My fingers were clumsy and slippery. I was sweating from every single pore in my body.

This must have been how that egg felt when it was right on the edge of its untimely demise.

Fuck it. Let's go.

"All right, hold ventilations and disconnect the vent."

The respiratory therapist manager followed the instructions. As soon as the vent was disconnected, I slipped the serpentine telescope into the breathing tube and dived down until I reached its end. Although to that point I had never seen the inside of a trachea, I had a strong suspicion that what I was seeing was not it. The firm, sturdy tracheal walls were nowhere to be found, and I surely wasn't seeing the fistula that was at the core of this issue. My scope was definitely inside a tube of some sort, but the walls were soft and mushy, undulating with rhythmic waves.

It was the inside of the sour straw candy. The tube had moved and gone completely through the fistula, and all of the oxygen that was meant for her lungs was being pumped into her esophagus. And her esophagus was trying to swallow the tube.

The descending chromatic scale of the oxygen monitor began to fall rapidly. We must have been down to about 60 percent. Come on, Chin-Quee.

I slowly pulled both the breathing tube and the scope backward, watching the slimy, muscular walls of the esophagus slide past my field of vision until suddenly I *popped* into a very different looking tube. This one was wide open, the walls sturdy and immobile, and in the distance I could see it split in two with one arm headed left and one headed right. I'd fallen into the trachea. And just past the tip of the breathing tube was a large hole connecting the trachea to the esophagus.

The oxygen monitor's melodic beeps had dropped five more times. Fifty-five percent. Somewhere far off in the distance I heard voices asking if I could see the problem, wondering if there was any way we could connect the vent again quickly, remarking that the sats were in the fifties. The voices in the room faded away. It was just me, my oxygen music, and the plumbing.

The silence was welcome, because I needed to solve a puzzle. I couldn't leave the tube where it was now—we would run into the same problem we'd had twenty minutes ago, and that would equal not enough oxygen. I also couldn't just push the tube in again, as there was nothing stopping it from just plunging through the fistula into the esophagus again. Without something to guide the tube down past the hole, this lady was going to be in deep—

Hold up. I was holding something to guide the tube in my hand already. My *scope* could be the guide.

Forty-eight percent. If this didn't work, I didn't know what else I would do.

I plunged my scope as far down the trachea as it would go, just past the huge hole, and then, using my free hand, I slowly pushed the breathing tube. For a sickening moment the tube refused to move, as if it were caught on something stubborn. Then, mercifully, the resistance gave way, and it slid down quickly and easily past the scope's tip, coming to a stop just above the right-left split. I removed the scope, held the tube in position, connected the vent tubing with my free hand, and nodded at the respiratory therapist. The ventilator switched back on and the chest rose and fell in mechanical tempo once more. I looked up at the monitor: 40 percent. I'd let her drop way too low.

The room waited in silence for several seconds, all eyes on the oxygen monitor. Five seconds passed. Then seven. At nine seconds, the number ticked up to 45 percent. It continued to rise steadily every two seconds until it reached 96 percent. The melody of the oxygen saturation monitor was high-pitched and monotonous— music to my ears. I taped the tube in place, thanked everyone in the room for their help, and walked/limped out into the hallway.

I found a nearby nurses' station and collapsed into a desk chair. Head in my very moist palms, I thought to myself: *I've officially sweated through three layers of clothing, including my white coat; my right ankle probably needs medical attention; I saved that lady's life; and I hate eggs.*

Kenny arrived ten minutes later. I quickly gave him the recap.

"Oh, wow, nicely done," he began. "But hey, did you get a sense of how far down the trachea the fistula is?"

"Uh . . ."

"Because that would have been really helpful. Oh, and did you get a sense of how big the fistula is in centimeters?"

"I, um . . . yeah, I'm not sure."

Kenny heaved an exasperated sigh. "All right. Just try to pay attention to things like that in the future. It'll help planning of the surgical intervention. We're going to go to the OR right now, so I'll call you when we're done and let you know how it goes." Within minutes the patient was whisked away.

I continued to sit for a few minutes as I wrestled with what had just happened. I'd been alone and in over my head. I'd somehow figured out and temporarily fixed a problem that could have killed someone. But I hadn't done it well enough. I hadn't paid attention to several things that I hadn't even been asked to pay attention to. And because of that, there would be no pats on the back, no kudos. Just keep working. Nine more hours.

The only thing I knew for sure? At the end of that day I was going to need a drink.

THREE

B-SIDE—THE FALL

Track 1: MY VOIS

It's been about a year since I've written anything that didn't end up in a patient's chart so . . . sorry, I guess. Been busy.

Yeah, it's most certainly been awhile. It's funny—you're able to find time for plenty of other things outside of work. Just not this.

Dude, I know. I just said I was sorry, and I'm here now, so what more do you want from me? I was procrastinating. Not the biggest deal in the world.

You're right. Sometimes, but . . . have you ever noticed that, for you, procrastination has always been an early sign of—

Enough of whatever it is you're trying to do here. I've got to purge this day from my body, so can I please just . . .

Yes. You can. Pour it all out.

Thank you.

Okay, so.

Freddy.

Yesterday I sat in a chair next to Freddy's hospital bed. The afternoon sun glinted off his long silver hair, giving a warm glow to the gown hanging from his slender frame. He huddled over a notepad, lips moving as he sounded out each letter. Freddy was sixty years old and had been born with a developmental delay. He'd been told that he reads and writes at a sixth-grade level. This might have been a bit generous.

Freddy also had a large cancer in his voice box. He required a *total laryngectomy*—a complex operation in which we would remove his entire voice box, pull up his trachea, and sew it into his skin, leaving him with a gaping hole in the front of his neck for the rest of his life.

He would never breathe air through his nose or mouth again. Without air passing through the nose, his sense of smell would decrease drastically. Without a sense of smell, food would never taste the same. Freddy loved french fries. Not for long—they'd likely taste like crispy cardboard after we were done with him.

Speech would require mastery of a small device that would make him sound like a robot. That or he'd have to learn how to belch his speech through his esophagus. Either option required a *lot* of teaching and a *lot* of practice. All to create a replacement voice that most people wouldn't be able to understand through their confusion / horror / asshole snickering. Freddy loved to sing along to the radio. He'd never hear his own voice again.

Oh, and he could never go swimming again. I had no idea if Freddy even liked to swim, but if he tried, he would flood his lungs within seconds and drown.

I worried for Freddy. We needed his permission to perform the surgery, and with no family to discuss it with, the decision was his alone. He was legally competent to make all of his own decisions, but the life-changing ramifications of what was to come were challenging for *me* to grasp, and I was the one with the medical degree. So I sat by his side that afternoon, spending minutes I didn't have to spare reviewing with him everything that would and could happen. As I spoke, I searched his hopeful eyes for any sign that he bore the true emotional weight of what was to come.

"Freddy, do you understand what's happening to you tomorrow?"

He could no longer speak due to the size of the tumor. His whispers were useless—he would run out of air after saying just two or three words. So I handed him a pen.

He labored over five words for two whole minutes, lips silently wagging, each stroke of ink carefully placed.

He handed the notepad back to me.

YOU HAVTA TAK MY VOIS.

I deflated with a sigh.

"Yeah, buddy. We have to take it."

He signed the consent.

This morning, just hours after he signed the paperwork, we ripped his voice box out of his neck.

Just another routinely devastating surgery.

After work this evening, I sat alone at a bar making condensation rings with the bottom of my beer glass, lost in increasingly hazy thoughts. Of course we had removed Freddy's cancer. Cancer is bad. That's Medicine 101. So by that logic, cutting the cancer out was . . . good, right? It had to be. *We'd done a good thing.* So why couldn't I shake the feeling that we had betrayed him?

I took a long sip from my glass. Then another. Freddy was a simple man. A happy man, but one with a simple understanding of the world's complexities. I knew in my heart that he didn't fully grasp the repercussions of the surgery—there was nothing simple about it. But surgery was what he needed to keep living, so we did it anyway because, according to a bunch of smart people who didn't know him personally, a life of any form or quality was better than no life at all. *We know what's best. We promise. So here, sign this consent form and give us control over your body.*

Was that not a betrayal of Freddy's trust and confidence? Did we truly "do no harm"?

And with that, I was awash with shame. Who was I to continue assuming that he didn't get it? Was I truly so elitist and judgmental that I "knew in my heart" that a grown man wasn't smart enough to take care of himself and make his own decisions because he crudely spelled words out phonetically?

My beer glass spun in my fingers as I grappled with the arrogant paternalism inherent in what I was being taught to do every day. *We know what's best.* We know our patients' bodies better than they do because we've studied the anatomical connections. We know their minds better than they do because we understand the chemistry that drives the brain. We shape their decisions and craft their self-interests in the image of our own because we are *so sure* that if they knew all that we know, they'd say yes to our recommendations without a second thought.

But what if my understanding of self-interest was a distorted, warped mess? My method of self-preservation was spending a Tuesday night getting drunk alone at the bar of a suburban Detroit Chili's. If the bartender were to offer me a bag of weed right there at the counter, I'd smoke that shit down and convince myself that getting behind the wheel of my car was fine because I wasn't technically "driving drunk." If the keyed-up business bro on the stool to my right told me that he had cocaine to share, I'd sniff it in the bathroom without hesitation, party with him till dawn, and still make it to rounds at 6:00 a.m. If someone, anyone, offered to keep me company in my bed tonight, I'd slip them my address. Saying yes to anything even slightly adventurous felt urgent these days. Almost a necessity, given my daily interactions with patients who'd been stripped of all agency.

Or maybe that's just my latest weak-ass justification for all of the dumb shit I've been doing with my free time.

And *that's* who knew best for Freddy. Some asshole who pre-served himself by pushing his luck until it inevitably ran out.

How could I possibly know what was best for someone else when I was nowhere close to knowing what might destroy *me*?

The thought nearly made my stomach turn. I got ahead of it by quickly downing the rest of my beer. I ordered another before my glass hit the counter.

It's been a year of this shit. A year of making decision after life-changing decision for people who were so desperately vulnerable in their illnesses that they could barely speak for themselves. And a year of my sorry-ass drinking by myself in busy public spaces so that I could maintain the flimsy belief that at least I wasn't drink-ing alone. Because if I were, then I'd be a dude with a problem in-stead of what I still hope I am—a kid trying to cope with having too many questions and never enough answers.

I unfolded a piece of paper from my pocket, smoothed it on the bar, and studied Freddy's penmanship. All capital letters written by an unsure hand. I snapped a photo. It felt worth remembering.

Then I raised my glass.

Here's to your vois, Freddy. I hope we did the right thing.

Track 2: ASH(Y)

Detroit winters are long.

Daylight is in short supply, and the sky is often a suffocating shade of gray. The forecast usually calls for either snow or the threat of snow. Everyone loves the initial snowfalls, but the novelty quickly wears off once the reality of living in a real-life *Frozen* sets in on your way to work. Chipping away at the ice on the windshield, knowing that it portends black ice on the pavement of the I-75 freeway, and saying a quick prayer for your lack of both tire tread and four-wheel-drive capability stops being cute after the first three weeks of the season. And in Detroit, winter generally lasts from the end of October through March.

In the 7:00 a.m. darkness of a Saturday morning in January, I sat in my little Japanese sedan on the street outside my apartment building, uselessly pumping the gas pedal as my wheels spun helplessly against a wintry mix of snow and ice. I put the car in park, sat back, and watched the fog of my deep sigh fill the frigid air around me.

This place was sucking my life force.

I was just starting my weekend on call but had been at work the night before until 9:00 p.m. assisting with a surgery. I'd slumped into my ice-cold apartment soon thereafter, immediately wrapped myself in a blanket, and ate half a plate of takeout Thai. With each howl of the wind, a piercing whistle of air rushed through the masking tape I'd placed over a fist-size hole in a windowpane. The hole had been there since before I'd moved in. The apartment actually had a history of gaping holes—the previous tenants had used the place as a set for low-budget porn films.[1] My landlord gave me a deal on the rent due to the place's colorful history and promised to fix the window quickly. It'd been eighteen months. Because Detroit.

And now my radiator was broken. In fucking January.

My last thought before drifting off into a fully clothed, blanket-cocooned sleep on my couch was that the upside of being in a thirty-degree apartment was that I didn't need to break the heat seal of my comforter to put the rest of my Thai food in the fridge. I was living in a motherfucking igloo. It was Coffee Table as a Fridge Friday in my living room, and the thought warmed my cold, dead heart.

My pager jolted me awake a few restless hours later. I was to report to one of our satellite hospitals in the Detroit suburbs as soon as possible. Something about a teenager . . . couldn't breathe . . . not sure if a breathing tube will fit . . . mounting panic . . . send help . . . the information came too quickly for my sleeping brain to handle. Nonetheless, I threw my blanket off, shoveled table-refrigerated pad see ew into my mouth, and was out the door in a matter of seconds, only to find myself in a car-shaped metal box with useless spinning wheels, sabotaged by winter.

Plus, waves of nausea were crashing through my body.

The table refrigerator was a bad choice.

Fifteen minutes of dry heaves and desperate shovel work later I was driving/ice-skating up the freeway to the hospital. I met my attending, Dr. Lopez, in the lobby and did my best impression of someone who was well rested, showered, and totally not wearing the same scrubs and sweaty underwear as yesterday.

A smile bloomed across his face. As our resident hipster faculty

---

1. Trust me, there is a *lot* you'll overlook in order to find a place with affordable rent. I'd decided that the porniness of my apartment was only gross if I thought about it too much.

member, he could always be counted upon to introduce me to the styles in vogue with the beard-worshipping, organic-urban-farm-cultivating, basement-bathtub-beer-brewing cool kids of Detroit. This morning he'd gone with horn-rimmed glasses, a short-sleeved plaid farmer's button-down, sky blue skinny jeans fastened with a thrift store belt, and purple Converse All Stars.

I smiled. I mean, sure, I smelled like a Thai restaurant dumpster, and my mother would have been appalled by my tragically nappy hair, ashy elbows, and general lack of soap work. But this dude had shown up to an emergency in purple Chuck Taylors. It might just end up being a good day.

"Doctor." He nodded.

"Doctor."

We continued at a brisk walk toward the intensive care unit as I broke down for my attending the scene that would likely await us in a few moments: an eighteen-year-old female with a history of asthma and recurrent tracheal stenosis[2] who had been admitted two days earlier for difficulty breathing. She was being treated for a bad asthma attack, but this morning the medicines had stopped working, and there was concern about placing a breathing tube because of her history of problems in her trachea. The anesthesiologists requested our help in managing the airway.

Whaddayaknow? My brain *was* working this morning despite being half-asleep when I answered that phone call. Hot diggity.

We walked quickly through the dimly lit waiting area toward

---

2. *Stenosis* is a medical word for "narrowing." Thus, tracheal stenosis is an abnormal narrowing of the windpipe, which tends to result in difficulty doing things like breathing and staying alive. Both asthma and tracheal stenosis are disorders that narrow parts of the airway and result in a low-pitched, abnormal breathing noise called wheezing. Asthma can be treated with medications. Stenosis has to be surgically corrected. And this teenager suffered from both of these conditions, sometimes simultaneously. I'm sure you can see the challenge here. Hooray for plumbing, amirite?

the double doors leading into the ICU. The space was empty, save for one family—no doubt my patient's family—huddled in a corner near the frosted windows: a mother, a father, and four preteen siblings. I locked eyes with the parents for a moment as I passed, and to my surprise I didn't find fear in their gazes. Only exhaustion. I could tell that they'd been in seats just like these far too many times awaiting news about their daughter. With four other children to look after, there was only the slimmest possibility that restful sleep had come to either of them for months, perhaps years.

I turned away and pushed through the doors.

There was no need to search for the room number—down the hall to our left, nurses and assistants were buzzing in and out of one patient's room in particular. Two doctors huddled just outside the room speaking in hushed tones. One was tall and barrel-chested, with thick, slicked-back, uniformly gray hair. His neck was craned forward and his rimless glasses hung low on his nose, just as I'd expect from someone who'd spent his entire life looking down on the world of nongiants. He wore the hospital's signature light blue scrubs, a fanny pack on the right hip, and a stethoscope fastened to the left—the unofficial uniform of the anesthesiologist. The other doc was short and skinny, just a touch too small for his white coat, which was too baggy around the shoulders. He had very young features despite his aggressively receding hairline. As he nodded his head, his entire body followed, giving the impression that he was repeatedly bowing to the taller doctor throughout their conversation. This was the medical intensivist, the doctor who oversaw all of the patients in the ICU.

Relief flooded their faces once they saw us approaching. Dr. Tall approached Dr. Lopez. Dr. Small hung back, staring anxiously into the patient's room.

"Thanks for coming, guys," Dr. Tall began, pushing his glasses a bit farther up his nose. "You up to speed with this kid?"

We nodded.

"Great. So she started decompensating about an hour ago, as the asthma treatments stopped working. Her oxygen sats are in the mideighties right now, so we've got to get a breathing tube down, but I have no idea how far down or how narrow her stenosis is, so I wanted to have you guys here before we tried anything."

Dr. Lopez peered thoughtfully into the patient's room. Like me, he was listening through the commotion for the rhythmic chirp of the patient's oxygen monitor. The steadily developing pitch-matching software in my brain agreed with Dr. Tall: the oxygen saturation was likely around 85 percent. Dr. Lopez turned back to Dr. Tall.

"Do you think we should try this in the operating room instead of doing it right here?" Dr. Lopez asked. "We'd have a bit more control over the situation, and we'd have a lot more tools at our disposal."

"I'd love to. But I don't think she's stable enough to make it over there," Dr. Tall replied firmly. "If she tanks while we're on the way there, we'll be in major trouble."

Dr. Lopez regarded him thoughtfully for a few moments, chewing the inside of his cheek. Finally, he turned to me.

"Got a knife on you, doctor?"

I smiled. "I believe I do, doctor." Nowadays I never left home without one.

He turned back to Dr. Tall and nodded his agreement with the plan. Specifics were quickly discussed. Dr. Small would administer the drugs required to put the patient to sleep so that a breathing tube could be placed. Dr. Tall would attempt to place his longest

and skinniest breathing tube and squeeze it past the narrow segment of the trachea. He would have two chances to succeed. If he
was unsuccessful, Dr. Lopez and I would cut into the patient's
neck, find her trachea, slice it open, and place the breathing tube
in this manner.

The plan's simplicity was a requirement. Once we began, there
was no turning back. It could go wrong at any point, anxiety and
panic might set in, and disaster would threaten. But we would always come back to the plan. Chaos doesn't win if you stick to the
plan.

I jettisoned my white coat and pulled on a disposable plastic
gown and paper mask. The patient's room was abuzz with activity: two young nurses scurried to and fro, grabbing anything they
might need to assist Dr. Small; a balding respiratory therapist
firmly held a mask over the patient's face while he spoke quickly
with Dr. Tall. Adding to the cacophony were the chirps and beeps
of the vital signs monitor: heart rate 110; 20 breaths per minute;
oxygen saturation 84 percent.

I looked at the patient. I'll call her Luz. Luz was tall but heavyset, built like a wrestler. Her caramel skin glistened with sweat;
long black hair hung in a matted nest on her pillowcase. Despite
the noise of the room, the sound of her breathing pierced through
all—an agonizing screech escaped the depths of her chest every
three seconds. She seemed to be using every muscle in her body to
both pull in and push out each breath. Tears streamed from Luz's
eyes as she caught my gaze but, as with her parents, there was no
fear there. Even as she lay before me slowly suffocating, her eyes
were only exhausted.

I had to look away. Becoming a partner in Luz's despair was a
deviation from the plan that I could not afford.

"Okay, Luz, you're going to go to sleep now," said Dr. Tall as he bent low next to Luz's ear. He glanced up and nodded at Dr. Small, who began slowly injecting medications into Luz's IV. Within seconds awareness faded out of her eyes and her chest stopped rising. Her muscles were paralyzed. She could no longer breathe on her own.

Dr. Tall got to work. He bent low and placed an intubating scope into Luz's mouth. After a few moments, he held out his right hand and a nurse placed the breathing tube in his palm. He placed it quickly into Luz's mouth.

I stood on the right side of the bed, eyes closed, visualizing what Dr. Tall must be seeing. He'd placed his scope in the groove between the tongue and the epiglottis, then lifted toward the ceiling to expose Luz's vocal cords—the gateway to the trachea. He then slipped the breathing tube gently into her mouth, down her throat and through her vocal cords. The tube continued to slide easily down—

"Shit. I'm meeting some really firm resistance. Feels like it's at least two centimeters below the cords."

He rotated the tube in his hand a few times in an attempt to corkscrew through the blockage, but he couldn't get past. He'd found the stenosis. And it was narrower than we'd thought.

"Hand me the smaller tube," he said as he removed the failed breathing tube. The last few centimeters of the tube were covered in fresh blood. Not great.

Dr. Lopez assumed his position on the opposite side of the bed and looked over at me. I was already injecting numbing medicine into the front of Luz's neck. I stole a glance up at her oxygen saturation: 80 percent.

Dr. Tall was back into the throat with the second tube. After a moment he attempted his corkscrew maneuver again, with the same results. He was getting nowhere. Oxygen at 77 percent. Dr. Tall's time was up.

Dr. Lopez announced that we were going to cut the neck. Dr. Tall removed his scope from the patient's mouth and prepared his smallest endotracheal tube to give to us when the time came. I slipped a couple of towels under Luz's shoulders to help extend her neck, grabbed the scalpel blade with my right hand, and looked up at Dr. Lopez. He nodded. *Time to go to work.*

This procedure is called an emergency cricothyrotomy. It's the one that's always depicted in the movies: someone is choking in a restaurant and a Good Samaritan grabs a steak knife, slices into the person's neck, and then slips a sipping straw into their trachea. Life saved, day saved, and everyone high-fives, hugs, and makes out with each other. Super sexy.

For Luz, things were not sexy.

I plunged my knife into the midline of her neck, just below her Adam's apple, through skin, fat, and muscle in a "north to south" (not side to side) fashion, so as to avoid the major veins that run down the front of the neck. Some bleeding is expected. As I cut into Luz's neck, dark red blood erupted out of the incision like a geyser.

There shouldn't be this much blood, I thought. *There shouldn't have been a vein in the way. Something's not right.*

Stick to the plan.

Even with Dr. Lopez suctioning blood out of the wound, it was flowing too quickly for me to see into the hole. No matter. I didn't need to see. I stuck my left index finger into the incision and felt for the hard Adam's apple cartilage. Then I slid my finger slowly down to the end of the cartilage until I fell into a soft spot half the width of my fingernail. *Bingo.* My entry point.

I stole another glance up at the monitor. Oxygen sat: 68 percent. Heart rate: 140. Her body was panicking.

Holding my left index finger in place, I took my scalpel once again in my right hand. I laid the blade flush against my left finger and, using my finger as a guide, slid the knife down into the overflowing wound until I met resistance near the tip of my fingernail. I stabbed down decisively and cut from left to right, removed the knife, and poked my finger into the cut I'd just made. I was in the trachea.

Yes.

I held out my right hand and Dr. Lopez placed the breathing tube in my palm. I placed it into the bloody hole, following my left finger once again until I felt it slip into the trachea. I advanced it a couple of centimeters and felt it stop abruptly. The stenosis. I pushed and twisted the tube with as much force as I could muster. It would not go down. The oxygen monitor beeped at a low and ominous pitch. I looked up. *Twenty percent.* I adjusted my position, nearly climbing on top of Luz to get better leverage, and pushed the tube again. It would not budge. As her oxygen continued its melodic nosedive, I realized that I'd created a new, devastating problem—blood was now draining into her trachea through the tiny stenotic segment and into her lungs. Not only was she not getting any oxygen, she was drowning in her own blood.

An as-yet-unheard tone suddenly blared from the vitals monitor. No repetition or rhythm to this alert. Just a single, steady blare from the machine that nearly drowned out all others.

Luz's heart had stopped beating.

My hands froze. I looked up from the gushing neck at the stunned faces around me. For a moment, there was no movement in the room as we held a collective breath. My eyes found Dr. Small, who I'd honestly forgotten was in the room. He stood by the door, arms folded, his oversize coat bunched up around his neck, giving him the look of a clean-cut, balding hunchback. He caught my eyes, sucked in a deep breath, and stood up straight for the first time all morning.

As it turned out, he wasn't actually that small.

He began shouting out orders, assigning tasks. One nurse ran out of the room to fetch emergency medications to be injected. Another scrambled for paperwork with which to record all of the actions from this point on. From my perch on the patient's bed, my job was clear: chest compressions. I laid one hand on top of the other and clasped my fingers. Elbows straight, hands on the middle of the sternum, bend from the waist and push the upper body's weight into the chest, just as I'd learned in medical school. Dr. Lopez took over attempts to force the breathing tube into the bloody hole in Luz's neck.

This is the dreaded "code blue"—the protocol that is engaged when a patient's heart and lungs stop doing their jobs. The goal is to reestablish the ABCs: airway, breathing, and circulation. Without any one of these, resuscitation will not succeed. Luz's airway was blocked, and Dr. Lopez was having no better luck getting a breathing tube in place than I had. With the airway blocked, oxygen couldn't get to the lungs. Without oxygen from the lungs, the blood that I was forcing through the heart to the rest of the body with my compressions was useless.

Luz's body was dying.

I felt a cascade of snaps beneath my hands as her ribs gave way under my weight.

I kept pushing.

A new voice barked out orders. I looked up and saw Dr. Tall organizing the nurses, preparing injections, checking with Dr. Lopez on his progress. Dr. Small had disappeared. As the intensivist, running the code was his responsibility. Where the hell had he slipped away to?

Fuck it. I kept pushing.

My lower back burned. Sweat fell in streams from my forehead onto my glasses. The veins in Dr. Lopez's wiry arms popped with strain as he made another desperate attempt with the breathing tube. And then a low, guttural wail pierced the air.

I looked up to the door and found Dr. Small standing there. Luz's father was by his side, collapsing against the side of the doorway. Dr. Small was trying to say something to the man but was drowned out by another primal roar. Luz's father couldn't take his eyes off his daughter. She was unrecognizable: throat slit, face bathed in blood. He bellowed and wept at the sight of the massacre. Dr. Small strained to pull the man to his feet and then quickly led him out of the room.

"Everybody stop!" Dr. Small shouted as he stepped back into the room moments later. The room went silent, save the steady tonal reminder of Luz's still heart from the monitor. A nurse reached up and switched off the sound.

"The family has decided to stop all efforts to resuscitate. Time of death: nine thirteen a.m."

A funny thing happened to me in that moment as I regarded the balding senior physician, who had returned to his natural deferential posture. To that point in my training, I'd already learned one of the most valuable lessons: attending physicians were supposed to be examples of the type of doctor that I wanted to be. But, more important, they could also often be examples of the type of doctor I did *not* want to be. When they made mistakes, or were rude to their coworkers, or were standoffish with patients, I didn't like it, but I could understand how they'd gotten there. Each moment that we navigate throughout each day is shaped by innumerable past experiences, as well as the handful of priorities that vie for our attention in the present. No casual act of neglect or cruelty or simple bad judgment existed in a vacuum—there was a world of memories, pressures, and emotions that crafted each and every decision and interaction. So more often than not, I'd been able to choose compassion when my bosses fucked up. Because I knew that, given the right (or wrong) circumstances, the doctor I didn't want to be *could be me.*

What Dr. Small had done, however, was something very different. He'd had the responsibility to update the family on Luz's condition. He'd told them that her heart had stopped, that we had commenced CPR, but that it was unlikely to be successful. Perhaps her father had asked if he could come into the room, perhaps Dr. Small had offered to let him see her—I never did learn the truth. The bottom line was that Dr. Small was the gatekeeper of this bloody scene and, knowing full well what lay ahead, had waved Luz's father in to witness the last moments of his daughter's life— blood pouring from her neck and bubbling out of her mouth, face and lips blue, eyes rolled up in their sockets, body flailing like a rag doll as a stranger pushed his entire weight into her broken, flattened chest. An undignified, chaotic, inhumane nightmare, now seared into his mind for the rest of his days.

My mind raced in search of the reasoning behind what the fuck Dr. Small could have been thinking. Maybe he thought he was being compassionate? Perhaps letting Luz's father see the code would quickly convince him that further attempts to bring her back to life would only result in more brutality? Or maybe Luz's dad had been an asshole to Dr. Small every time she'd been admitted to the hospital, and this was a final "fuck you" to an intrusive and overbearing family member. Or maybe this was Dr. Small's version of giving Luz's family full autonomy—it would have been unethical for him to influence the decision to withdraw care with his own words, so better to allow Luz's father to make an informed decision with every last bit of bloody supporting evidence.

But whatever his reasoning, *he didn't fucking have to give this poor father this nightmare.* If he'd thought for one second beyond his own heartless agenda, he'd have realized that this decision could have been made back in the quiet calm of the family waiting area. He could have kept a vulnerable man safe from the horrors that, for us, have become routine.

Instead, he'd chosen cruelty. It wasn't spur of the moment. It was calculated. He'd chosen the wails. He'd chosen the harrowing scream.

And in that moment, as he called the time of death and slumped his defeated shoulders deeper into his oversize coat, I hated him for what he had done.

And there was nothing I could do to make it right.

I pulled off my bloody gown, gloves, and mask and trashed them as I rushed out of the room, eyes downcast. I spared no final glance at Luz, nor did I scan the hallway for her family. My pager needed tending to, and so I made straight for the nurses' station and began returning phone calls.

Within a few minutes, Dr. Lopez was by my side. He put a hand on my shoulder. I considered meeting his gaze. I thought about asking him if he'd seen what I'd seen. I wondered if he thought we'd made the right decisions. Instead, I sat in silence and made myself appear busy, scribbling nonsense notes on the papers in front of me.

"Hey," he said, "don't worry about the paperwork for this one. I'll take care of everything."

I nodded and quickly excused myself—there was a consult to see upstairs. I dipped into a stairwell and began a hurried climb to the third floor, only to stop at the first landing. I'd come upon an enormous window overlooking suburban Detroit: a low-hanging gray sky backlit by a sun that I was unlikely to see for several days, lording over cascading mounds of ice and snow. Stray snowflakes billowed about as the wind gusted and howled against the frozen glass. And then there was stillness. Silence. It rooted my feet to the ground. It wrapped its fingers around my throat. And squeezed.

Frenzied thoughts shot back and forth between my ears in a voice I just barely recognized as my own.

I hope her quinceañera was a good one, because that's probably the last great party she'd ever had. Because she's dead now.

You don't have to punish yourself. Just take a breath and slow—

I hope they had good cake. Maybe that was her last thought before I slit her throat. Funfetti and frosting.

Your mind is getting loud and overheated. Please try and—

I really hope she had sex with someone before today. You really shouldn't die before you know what that feels like. How do you have sex when you're always afraid that you're going to suffocate? Is that how she felt every day? "Is today the day that I just won't be able to breathe?"

You know her trachea was a ticking time bomb. No matter how many times she was temporarily fixed, this was going to be

the problem that killed her at some point. Today was . . . just her time.

Just her time. Were you even paying attention? We set the timer on that bomb this morning. We _made_ it her time. Our fucking plan. It was flawed from the beginning. We were ill-equipped. Not ready. Maybe if we'd had more time.

Trust me. Don't go down this—

Maybe if Dr. Lopez had spoken up more forcefully. Maybe if Dr. Tall wasn't so fucking tall. Maybe if Dr. Small wasn't such a goddamn feeble sack of shit. Maybe if I hadn't drowned her in her own blood while she was already suffocating.

You didn't kill—

Yes. I. We. _All of us_ killed this girl.

And if you'd done nothing? She'd have died anyway.

And that's supposed to, what, comfort me? Great fucking job. A+. Let's see, what else is comforting? How about the fact that I don't cry anymore? A child, a fucking _kid_, is dead. I helped kill her with my own hands. Her family is somewhere in this building in massive pain. And I can't cry because my brain is fucked. Always has been. Faulty wiring, right? And now the wires are splitting and fraying and sparking and dangerous and something might catch fire and explode and—

It's okay. Listen to me. It's okay to feel—

You are not listening. That's the problem, can't you see? I can't . . . fuck, look, I _know_ this is sad. I want to _feel_ sad. I used to feel . . . I want to feel this loss. Please.

Stay with me. Don't tip over the edge.

Loss. Pain. Fear.

If you fall, I won't be able to follow. You can still find—

Loss. Lost.

Lost.

Please don't tell me I'm already lost.

Is that someone giggling at me?

Don't listen. You ca . . . trust . . .

Who's there? Why can't you leave me to scream in my silence? Two more hearty cackles? Three? Four? THIS IS NOT FU—

The wind howled again, shaking the window and jolting me back to the world outside my head.

I was not okay. Probably losing my fucking mind. But this job, this place . . . It couldn't care less.

One deep breath, then I turned and continued up the stairs.

I arrived at the next patient's door. The day was just beginning, the halls filled with nurses chatting about their patients, weekends, and children as they rounded. A normal Saturday on the ward. I buttoned my coat, knocked twice, and reached for the handle. As I took the first step through the threshold, something caught my eye: my left shoe. Luz's blood had dripped all over it, and it was now dark, dried, and sticky. My shoe was black. The only one who'd know the blood was there would be me. And I couldn't bring myself to clean it.

My mind drifted again—it's been getting more and more difficult to stay present lately—this time to a recent memory. Two weeks ago, I was walking down a suburban street outside Detroit when the sight of the skeletal, burned-out remains of a home suddenly arrested my progress. There had been a fire mere days before, and the smell of charred timber still hung thick in the air despite the recent snowfall. The ghostly plot was a blight on the neighborhood's pristine facade. Any passersby instinctually gave the place a wide berth. I approached.

I checked the mailbox, respecting its tenuous hold on the fallen, warped doorframe. Empty. I crossed the front door's threshold, treading carefully through the signs of a disrupted life that peeked through inches of snow—here a shred of a knitted blanket; there a participation trophy for a youth soccer league; framed photographs of tropical landscapes scattered along a carpeted staircase that led to a nonexistent second story; the singed mirror of an antique vanity. I ran my fingers over it. *Someone used to live here.* There had been warmth and comfort, laughter and loss. There had been love here. And it had all burned. I stood amid the bones of that house until my toes cried out for respite from the cold.

I've been wandering a lot lately. Always in the cold. Sometimes in the dark. Never giving nearly enough thought to why the city's desolate, broken things have been drawing me in.

Until this confusing, bloody moment on the gray morning of Luz's death.

I used to feel feelings. Feel them in the way I believe most people do: by accident. The big, broad emotions—happiness, anger, fear, pain—I took them all for granted. I never really interrogated them because they were baked into me at birth. Like the five senses, our basic emotions are quite simply part of what it means to be human. I never had to question how to feel them—they just happened naturally. Unfortunately, by that same measure, I never learned how to retrieve them should they ever get lost.

And I'd lost them. I'd been slowly and steadily betrayed by the truth of this profession, my faulty survival instincts, an increasing inability to control my own thoughts, and left with nothing but ash where those pieces of my humanity used to be. And I'd barely noticed. Those feelings had been born so strong, loud, and passionate. But when they turned fragile, they burned away silently. Insidiously.

Until the sight of Luz's blood on my left shoe, invisible to all but me, finally brought my deficiencies to light. Wow, what a psychological breakthrough. All it took was the act of killing a kid. If a school bus blows up tomorrow and bits and pieces of children roll into the emergency room, I might be able to put myself through the equivalent of years of free therapy.

A well-adjusted sentiment if there ever was one.

Fuck. Pitch-black thoughts about dead kids. This might be all I have left.

Because it had all burned. And the hope that there was still something in this house left to salvage would set me on nothing but a fool's errand—the death rattle of a man who'd long since forgotten the depth of agony and the catharsis of tears.

Someone used to live here.

Already lost.

I pushed open the patient's door.

"Good morning, ma'am. I'm Dr. Chin-Quee. So I hear you fell and bumped your nose?"

Track 3: HANDS

I met a lady a month ago. I was one of several doctors crowding around her and her husband in a claustrophobic clinic exam room. Standing silently for fifteen minutes as my bosses droned on about serious medical stuff, I barely heard a word as I fought a rising unfamiliar and unprofessional compulsion. As the doctor parade filed out, I just couldn't hold it in any longer.

I asked if I could photograph her. Just her hands. Her fingers, actually. I knew it was weird. Completely unrelated to what she had come into the clinic for but . . . would she mind? She raised her eyebrows warily. She needed to hear some noncreepy reasoning for this clearly nonmedical request. Of course she did. And, of course, I found myself completely inarticulate. I had no idea why her hands were calling out to me. Only that I needed to listen. And there was no way to say that in a way that wouldn't freak her out. My lips silently wrapped around the beginnings of dozens of explanatory words until she mercifully held up a hand, then extended it toward me.

"Just promise me you'll make something beautiful with it," she said.

I've stopped and started writing about her so many times that I think it's time to accept that the words are desperate to come out in another way.

I'm smart enough to know that I'm no great poet.

But sometimes verse feels like the only way through.

You sat next to your husband under the humming fluorescent
    lights,
Linoleum beneath your feet.
The room was all right angles
And there was stillness in the urban tundra just beyond the
    window
The moment we told you that your cancer had returned.

This time it would be the death of you.

Shoulders back, head high, eyes placid pools.

Had you known all along that the journey would lead here?
Or had you simply decided long ago that
        Should you lose,
            There would be dignity in the moment?

Either way, I believed you.
Most of you.

Your left hand hung by your side, a study of stillness

Until a single muscle jumped.
Soon twitched another
And another.

Each finger writhed and swayed and cried out in its own
      cadence

Individual serpentine dances of despair and desperation
Punctuated by rigid extensions of panic and limp falls of
      defeat
And just as tension crept into the nest of tendons around your
      wrist, portending the spread of the sickness

There was his hand, fallen from its perch.

His fingers sprang to life.
Never grazing your skin.
He knew all of the spaces in between
And caressed them gently, purposefully
Guided by decades of study,
            a pupil of the unnamed spaces that shape you.

Your fingers slowed

Then stopped
Then closed, wrapping delicately around each of his.
            They were exactly where you knew they'd be.

Your eyes, his eyes,

They never left us.
Your bodies betrayed no knowledge of the conversation
   between your hands.
And as we described the shape your death would take,
I wished selfishly
That someone, someday, might know my negative space.
A silent prayer that there would be one who embraced the
   weight of my silences,
      Knew the depths of my shadows
         And could dance in all of my spaces in between.
Before I am gone.

I folded my arms across my chest

To protect against the chill that came from knowing:

      I was never any good at prayers.

*T*his is the first time in a long, long time that you've created
   something like this.

I'd love to say that that fact is comforting, but . . .

She wanted me to honor her. And all I did was make it about
me. As usual.

*Well, she wasn't your muse. She was just the vessel for what's
been keeping you up at night: your desire for connection, and all
of the meaningful shapes it might take. Once you let that in, your
pen couldn't write fast enough.*

Yeah. I don't know. It feels like all I was able to do was get way
more articulate about how fucking lonely I am. And it feels . . .

Maybe I'm better off not searching for the art hidden in all of these moments anymore.

Track 4: BED TIMES—LIVE FROM THE SHEETS

"So, I've got to tell you. The fact that you and I have the same name is a complete, dual-cheek pain in my ass."

I glanced at the rearview mirror. Hints of gray had been creeping into my hair. My cheeks had gotten a bit rounder underneath my beard stubble. My eyes tended to squint a bit when I searched for words.

My father's features.

They'd been sneaking in over the last few years, hadn't they? Apropos that I was finally able to see them for what they were in that instant, as my father sat in the passenger seat to my right.

He remained silent.

I remained furious.

"I mean, did you ever stop for a second to think about what might happen when debt collectors couldn't track you down?" I continued, my voice rising. "They fucking called *me*. I'm as close to you as they could get. And I just kept telling them that I didn't know where you were or how to contact you."

My eyelids hung heavy as the scenery adorning I-75 whipped past the windshield. This man had a way of exhausting me.

"I should have just told them," I spat with barely subdued rage. "Where has loyalty to you ever gotten me? What has believing in you ever fucking gotten me? Disappointment, old man. Every fucking—OH MY GOD, NO, I DON'T WANT ANY GOD-DAMN COTTON CANDY!"

He had pushed a handful of pink cotton candy next to my face—a silent, insistent peace offering. It was 9:30 a.m. I was driving home from work after a night on call and I was starving. Of course he *would* try to feed me cotton candy. It wouldn't sustain me. Ain't no vitamins in that shit.

"Are you even listening?! I can't buy a car. I can barely get an apartment. I can't take out loans because my credit is trash. Because they just gave me your debts when they couldn't find you. I keep getting punished because of you. And I haven't had the time to fight it because I'm just so—"

"Facials?"

We'd stopped at a light on Woodward Avenue. I glanced at him over the rims of my glasses, making sure I'd understood the first heavily accented word he'd said to me for the entire ride.

"You want to . . . go and get facials?" I asked.

"Facials," he repeated with Jamaican enunciation, nodding his head as if I'd finally figured out life's great mystery.

"I mean . . . I mean, yeah, that sounds . . . really refreshing."

I was suddenly having a lot of trouble remembering what I'd been angry about. We were going to be a couple of dudes having a nice father-son time at a day spa. Life wasn't all bad, was it?

"All you need to do is stop," he said calmly. "Stop moving. Stop rolling. Just stop."

"Dude, wait. Fuck the spa. I was saying something really—"

His face contorted in panic as he grabbed my shoulder, screaming,

"TONY, STOP!!!"

My eyes shot open as I crunched into the bumper of the car in front of me. I slammed my brakes, several seconds too late, and looked around my car wildly. The passenger seat was empty. Of course it was—I hadn't seen or spoken to my father in two years. I couldn't remember anything about the drive home from work.

I'd been asleep the entire time.

2:48 p.m.

My residency program director will henceforth be referred to as the General. He'd never, to my knowledge, served in the military. However, the precision of his buzz cut and razor-sharp flattop could be rivaled only by those disaster movie lieutenants who gruffly badger the president to input the nuclear launch codes and blast the Russians / aliens / planet-destroying asteroids to kingdom come. The unspoken rule among older residents was that you never spoke to the General unless spoken to, never looked him directly in the eye out of respect, and never questioned him, especially when he started breathing heavily through his nose.

Three hours ago I was called into his office. I had just finished a thirty-hour stint in the hospital, and various parts of my body were starting to fall asleep against my will. I slumped into a chair facing his desk—there would be no military-grade subordinate posturing today.

"You're over your duty hours again," he said in a soft, smooth baritone.

I shrugged. "Sounds about right." I found myself wondering if he had to apply product to his hair every day to get it to stand up so straight, or if he had one of those weird relatives who was a porcupine.

"You're the only resident who's consistently going over eighty hours a week." He punctuated his statement with a long nasal exhalation.

It finally dawned on me that he was a chronic loud nose breather. It didn't matter what mood he was in—he was always breathing loudly through his nose. He really should see a doctor about that. He probably knew that. The nose doctor knows he needs a nose doctor. Or was it that he *nose* he needs a nose doctor? Ha!

I chuckled at the comedic gold running through my head, and the General raised a questioning eyebrow. I was losing the thread of this conversation quickly. My brain was only barely awake.

"Yeah, boss. I really don't know why that is. We're all working the same call schedule. I'm pretty sure we should all be over our hours all the time."

"Well, when I look at the breakdown, the difference is that they are regularly logging hours off for sleep each night that they're on call, and you don't."

Well, shit. That'd do it.

"Well, shit, General. That'd do it." I shifted in my chair and pinched myself in the thigh. Pain keeps you awake. "I mean, I'm up all night seeing consults, writing notes, on the phone with nurses, doing all of the stuff I'm supposed to do. I only ever manage an hour of sleep, if that, each night I'm here."

"Well, you've got to find a way to get more efficient with your time," he said, leaning forward. "If the others can do it, so can you. If you keep going over your hours like this, we're going to start getting a bunch of phone calls from the ACGME, and the program could be in trouble."

The ACGME was the watchdog council that had mandated the eighty-hour resident workweek nearly a decade ago and held the power to shut us down if we were out of compliance. And because of me, they might start sniffing around, asking questions they didn't want to know the answers to. Of course it was *me* that was the problem. The program shouldn't have to suffer because I wasn't moving fast enough. "Can do, boss. I'll get more efficient."

I needed a snappy sign-off so that I could start inching closer to my bed across town.

"I'm going to get moving on home now. Thank you for your concern and stalwart leadership." I nearly tripped on the chair as I rose and backed out of the room. "Warmest regards. Best wishes. Godspeed. Sweet dreams, sir."

I made it home to my bed shortly thereafter and was soon dead to the world but woke shivering and disoriented two hours later—like a champ, I'd forgotten to turn on the (finally repaired) heat before I'd passed out. Brilliant. An unperturbed, pagerless sleep was one of the few parts of my life I looked forward to these days. Oh well, guess that plan is fucked for today.

So now I lay in bed, comforter pulled up to my nose, contemplating my third meeting with the General in as many months.

Get more efficient. I've heard that phrase over and over, not just from the General but from my senior residents as well. I think it stems from the unspoken and unofficial (but totally official) surgeon credo: *Do more work in less time. Because if you do eighty hours of work at normal speed each week, you'll only learn enough to be a glorified, high-tax-bracket butcher by the end of five years . . . Why are you crying? There is no salty eye discharge in surgery!* I think they all figure that the statement about efficiency will suffice as an all-encompassing piece of advice. Unfortunately, nobody seems to realize that "get more efficient" in isolation, without any specifics as to how to do it or any exploration into why I'm struggling to accomplish it, is nothing more than an admonishment. *Get more efficient = You're not trying hard enough.*

It really should be a simple problem to solve. I'm just as smart as my fellow residents. I can figure this out. Get the same amount of work done in significantly less time so that I can sleep. I could start by spending less time with patients and just rushing through conversations a bit more . . . I definitely have to write notes faster . . . Maybe I could get more of my computer work done outside the on-call room—having a bed right next to me as I worked was just making me sleepier . . . Plus, Amazon is supposed to deliver my teleportation ring in a couple of days. Free shipping. God bless Amazon Prime. What a time to be alive. And finally, I seem to recall a plan to supply each of us with a full-time on-call penguin assistant. A personal penguin by my side, just taking care of the paperwork. I know they look like they're wearing suits, but in the name of decorum, I'll probably push to have actual bird-size suits made for them. They're not savages, for God's sake . . .

Shit.

I fell asleep again.

This has been happening more and more often. Whether I sleep for two hours or nine, I always seem to wake up exhausted. It's likely because, on top of not sleeping often or long enough, I have a wonderful condition called obstructive sleep apnea. Folks with OSA try their best to go to sleep just like regular humans but are betrayed by their bodies as soon as they drift off. As they sleep, the anatomy of their throats—usually the tongue, tonsils, and soft palate (from which the uvula, the hangy ball in the back of your mouth, dangles)—collapses inward, blocking their airways. If you can force air past the blockage, you make a fun noise called snoring. If you can't force air past the blockage, it's called an apnea: you don't breathe because you're choking on your own throat. Then your body panics due to lack of oxygen and forces you to wake up so that you can voluntarily take a few deep breaths. I got tested for obstructive sleep apnea at some point in medical school and learned that in my sleep I hold my breath and go apneic about eighty-five times an hour. The levels of oxygen in the blood that reach my brain often dip so low that I can safely say I have the equivalent of several mild strokes any time I sleep. And that's been every night. For years. Of course, I want to get the necessary surgery, but I just never had the money or the time off—a surgery, coincidentally, that I've started learning to perform as an ENT resident.

So I don't get enough sleep at work because I'm not trying hard enough, and the sleep that I do get isn't restful because I choke myself all night. Then I wake up even more tired than I was before I slept, and my thoughts weave in and out of waking dreams throughout the day. And finally the combination of my pride and perceived isolation from my peers—their long sighs and eye rolls when I tell them of another sleepless night on call make how few fucks they give about me painfully clear—has resulted in an unwillingness to ask for help.

I'm just too tired to figure out how to be less tired.

Until I can get a handle on this, I know one thing for sure: I do not need the added stress of being known as the resident who took down the entire program because of excessive duty hours.

Starting tomorrow, I will commit to lying about my hours.

In the eyes of my program, I will never work more than eighty hours a week again.

And they'll totally buy it.

It's not their body suffering the consequences of toeing the party line, so why wouldn't they?

1:07 a.m.

In the words and vocal cadence of the forty-fourth president of the United States of America: *let me be clear*—doctors *absolutely* make more mistakes when they are tired. In these last several months of sleepless days and nights, I have routinely misread and misspoken, forgotten important details, and left tasks incomplete. The saving grace for my patients is that I rarely make mistakes in a vacuum—the rest of the team usually catches them before any harm comes to anyone. So this morning (or was it yesterday morning?) after I wrote my patient summaries while partially asleep and described a woman as "a fifty-six-year-old female with a history of pink surly elephant White Castle security monkey," my senior resident caught the error as we discussed on morning rounds, and neither animal control services nor the circus was called.

Unfortunately, outside the hospital I don't have the luxury of several people looking over my shoulder as I make questionable decisions. My ass should be asleep right damn now. Instead, I'm pounding a sack of White Castle cheeseburgers and trying to convince myself that I'll turn off the TV at the next commercial break, but honestly there's no way in hell that will happen because *Sister Act 2* is on, and if I'm not awake to witness these singing-ass urban youths winning the gospel choir competition, their happy ending won't actually happen.

Because left to my own devices, my judgment these days *rocks*.

Anyway, since I'm awake, I might as well take an awesome

inventory of my recent A+ life choices. Here's a short list of things forgotten, neglected, or just plain done wrong in my personal life during this time of peak sleep deprivation:

1. Food

The last thing I want to do once I leave the hospital is go food shopping, so I just . . . don't. I could probably count on two hands the number of times I've gone to the supermarket in the last two years, and half of those trips were to see if Kroger had a two-for-one sale on frozen pizza. To make matters even more troubling, a few months ago the hospital's twenty-four-hour Little Caesar's pizzeria was replaced by a twenty-four-hour Subway sandwich shop. I quickly convinced myself that it was a totally reasonable and healthy food option compared with pizza that had been genetically engineered to be both Hot-N-Ready while it sat on a shelf for twelve straight hours.[3] So on days that I'm on call, I regularly eat at Subway for four meals a day, each of which includes a complimentary large soda and extra chocolate chip cookies because the girls who work the register think I'm cute.

Vegetables come in the form of chopped iceberg lettuce and green peppers between rubbery pieces of bread; fruits in the form of lemonade and Cherry Coke. Needless to say, the *ellbees*[4] have begun to pile onto my previously wiry frame. Good thing scrubs help me maintain an air of mystery about my rapidly widening physique.

---

3. I believe in the miracles of science as much as the next guy, but ain't no way that pizza could be good for you. That science ain't sciencing right, you know?

4. Ellbees = LBs = pounds = extra trunk junk and handles of love.

2. Laundry

I have to pay to use the washers and dryers in my apartment building, so spending precious loose change to wash scrubs makes no sense to me. I get them free from the hospital, and I've long since figured out how to hustle the mechanical dispensers to give me as many sets as my heart desires. So I don't wash—I just get more. At any given time, I have twelve to fifteen sets of scrubs in a pile on my bedroom floor. And not one of them is clean.

I'm not anti–clean clothing. It's just that at some point I stopped remembering to allot the three minutes a day it would take to exchange my dirty scrubs for clean ones in the dispenser. So each morning I sniff the pile for the least offensive set and throw it on. Dirtball rationalization has led me to believe that as long as my underwear is (mostly) clean, and there isn't too much in the way of old blood or human secretions in plain view, nobody will ever know that I regularly wear scrubs that have not been washed in a calendar year.

And that is a conservative estimate.

Because my name is Tony. And I'm a dirtbag trash monster.

3. Bills

I'd love to be able to pay all of my bills in their entirety and on time. But I'm very often dead-ass broke. And not that cute "Oh, I've only got a few hundred in the bank, I guess I can't order the Emperor's Feast at Benihana" sort of broke. I'm talking about digging through an old coffee can for nonpenny loose change in order to scrape together enough to put a single gallon of gas in my car. Actual no-physical-money, state-of-perpetual-overdraft broke.

So how did I manage to find myself in a near-constant state of financial calamity? I'm pretty sure it's because nobody ever taught me how to manage money. Growing up, I was privy only to snippets of my family's troubled relationship with money: the mortgage was a hangman's noose, impassively tightening every month; my father only ever paid in cash, never had a credit card; my mother kept the family on a strict bottom-shelf-at-the-supermarket budget except for those two days every couple of months when she'd get intensely sad or angry and treat herself to such an extravagant credit card shopping spree that she'd force herself to snip the card in half the next day in shame; nobody ever had any savings or investments or markers of stability. I never learned how to plan. And it turns out that when you strike out on your own into different cities across the country with hundreds of thousands of dollars in debt, a maxed-out credit card, and a job that pays you the equivalent of minimum wage for the number of hours you put in, a plan is probably in your best interest.

Things I didn't plan for include: how much of my paycheck should go toward rent (definitely not 50 percent), how much of my paycheck would be garnished by taxes (a lot of percents), how a credit card bill will never change if all you can afford to pay is the monthly minimum (rude), and the extent to which people who send you bills every month actually want to be paid. Turns out they really want their money. Sadly, unless I've been paying close attention to the angrily stamped envelopes in my mailbox or the toll-free calls I tend to send straight to voice mail on one of the two days of the month I get paid, not enough increasingly impatient people will receive the payments they rightfully deserve.

And paying attention is not exactly my strong suit these days.

So I have no money plan, I can't keep on top of these bills because I'm so tired I might be going cross-eyed, and in the moments when I can grasp just how tumultuous my financial life is, I'm so ashamed of myself for not knowing better and panicked by the possible consequences that I just . . . stay awake when I should be asleep, eat sliders in front of the TV, and ultimately . . . do nothing about it.

But on the bright side, I have picked up a few nifty broke-boy tricks of the trade that help keep the lights on. For example, I've learned that if I've got a few cents in my checking account, I can still use my debit card to buy something way more expensive! Several Subway breakfast sandwiches have come from exploiting this surprising overdraft loophole. Delish. And since I get my phone and internet services from the same provider, I've found that when I don't pay for either one on time, it's the internet that usually gets turned off first. Thank God, because if my cell service got cut off, I'd be massively fucked at work. Losing internet service works great as a "pay your fucking phone bill" alarm.

I honestly have no idea what I'm going to do if all of this shit catches up to me.

Not sure if it's the sliders or the money talk, but I'm starting to feel a little queasy.

4. My Mom's Birthday

In my defense, I didn't *completely* forget that the woman who birthed me has a birthday. I just forgot which day it was. Actually, I wouldn't even go that far—I definitely knew which day it was. It's just that the date I was certain of turned out to be completely wrong.

On the day I thought was her birthday, I confidently called my mother to wish her well and was shocked to hear the disappointment in her voice as she answered the phone, exactly one day after her actual birthday. We had a brief argument about whether she was remembering her own birthday correctly, until she made me actually say the correct date out loud. December 3rd. I paused as the rusty gears in my brain started turning. *Hot damn, she might be right . . . about her own birthday.*

Such is life in the world of working hundred-hour weeks, suffocating in your sleep, and sweating Subway onion essence out of your pores into scrubs that haven't been washed since the end of Obama's first term.

I apologized for my diminished processing capacity. She said it was okay with a practiced, exhausted sincerity that made me feel even more hopelessly incompetent.

That's it, isn't it? That's how sleep deprivation really feels: hopeless.

Going months without a true night of sleep has left me at the mercy of all of the things my brain has lost the capacity to prioritize and organize, and it feels as if there isn't a damn thing I can do about it. I just keep opening my eyes each morning, whether I've slept or not, resigned to the expectation that some mess I've unwittingly made will come and bite me in the ass by nightfall.

If I had the energy, I'd let the embarrassment and humiliation of it all sink in.

I'd admit how disappointed in myself I am. All the fucking time.

But honesty is too taxing. It's way easier to laugh at how smelly and overweight and haphazardly constructed my deadbeat life has become.

Ah, the kids from *Sister Act* won first place. I knew they could do it.

10:18 a.m.

Instead of closing my eyes in search of sleep this morning, I've been dicking around on the internet. I came across this article that I can't stop reading. I've already been through it five times. It began by describing a young Black man who, by the age of twenty-nine, was both a YouTube singing sensation and a physician. Like me, he was a resident. He was training in the field of family medicine. Around the hospital he was known affectionately as "the Singing Doctor," a title bolstered by the fact that he'd once been invited to sing onstage with Boyz II Men and had successfully auditioned to be a contestant on *America's Got Talent*.

I found myself giving the Black Guy Head Nod to my laptop screen as I read. Young Black man with the smarts to doctor, the voice of a superstar, and the courage to be both? I see you, bro. Maybe clearer than most.

The article continued.

Shortly after his audition, a friend who had just worked a long shift (it's unclear if the friend was a health care professional) was giving him a ride from the hospital to a family event out of town. The friend fell asleep at the wheel, swerved off the highway and into a tree.

Brandon Rogers, the Singing Doctor, died shortly after the crash from injuries he'd sustained in the passenger seat. The driver survived.

It's here that I stop reading and begin again from the top. Then stop and restart again. Because I don't know why I'm not feeling what I think I should feel.

Brandon's death was a tragedy, right? An overwhelming tragedy.

At least it should feel that way. Especially to me. Because he *was* me. Though the journalist eulogized him with mentions of his most notable and public achievements, I can read between the lines. I know the weight of expectation that he'd carried. I know the ways in which he was made to feel both invisible and spotlighted in a profession that couldn't quite understand him. I know how much shit his colleagues must have spoken about him when they heard he'd auditioned for a singing show. And I know how strong the pull of music on his heart must have been to convince him that he had no choice but to surrender to it.

Now all of that passion, all of that success, and all of that potential is gone from this world. Brandon is dead.

Yet despite all of our similarities, I feel no connection to him. No sadness. Nothing.

But I'm not empty, as I've been feeling fairly often these days. My feelings of sympathy and empathy are there, it's just . . . they've taken an unexpected path: I am mourning his friend. His killer. The driver who lived.

I'm pretty sure he wishes he'd died in that crash too.

I know I would.

It's got to be easier to have the lights go out in an instant than to watch the life you knew disappear before your eyes, leaving you with nothing but darkness, ghosts, and whispers. That stain of taking someone's life . . . I've learned that it never washes clean. And it drags with it a chorus of silent whispers of regret, of self-flagellation, of *why*s and *what-if*s. For the rest of his life, the driver will convince himself that everyone around him asks behind his back the same torturous question he asks himself every day. Every hour.

If you were that tired, why did you get behind the wheel?

He may never know the answer. But I do.

The tragic truth is that humans tend to underestimate how tired they are. And that's through no fault of their own—it's an adaptive behavior performed by our brains. When we perform active tasks, we feel less tired, no matter how exhausted we are—the brain sees new challenges before it that require close attention and problem-solving, so it tricks itself into staying up and awake.

So the driver? He felt *fine* when he got into the car, fired up the ignition, pulled out, and charted the initial course of the ill-fated road trip. But once the task of driving got easy on the highway and demanded less active surveillance, his brain relaxed, just as it's wired to do. It happened in seconds. Before he could even register that he was tired, he was already asleep.

Even though I understand how it all works, the knowledge doesn't help me make better decisions.

Fun fact: My hospital has a program that reimburses residents for taxi rides if they are feeling too tired to manage the drive home after a long shift. Most hospitals with residents in training do. Unsurprising fact: Nobody uses that shit. We just don't feel dangerously tired as we go through the physical motions of leaving the hospital—just as our brains intend for us to feel. But we know the science. We totally know we're being tricked. Even so, we'll always do a quick calculus to rationalize the decision to drive—*I really don't live that far away! It'll be such a pain to come back and get my car later! The paperwork for the taxi reimbursement will take weeks!*—and driving always wins. So we leave the parking lot with the windows rolled down and the music on full blast to keep ourselves awake, even though we know that shit doesn't work. Once we've been in our cars for a few minutes on those familiar routes we drive every day . . . we might do things like have a nonsensical conversation with an estranged father.

And we might just punctuate that conversation by crashing into the car in front of us.

Just like I did an hour ago.

As it turns out, the only damage I did was a minor scratch to the other car's bumper. A middle-aged lady in a business suit hopped out of the driver's seat and met me behind her car. I apologized profusely, made up some story about hitting the wrong pedal with my foot, and she brushed the entire situation off with a good-natured midwestern laugh, wished me a good morning, and was on her way. I was home within the next five minutes.

That was my second car accident in as many weeks. Arriving home from work with no memory of the trip is becoming a dangerously common occurrence.

I'm a fucking public health hazard. And that's . . . suboptimal. A total big deal that I should, I don't know, reevaluate and do something about, but . . .

All I want to do is sleep.

So nighty night.

Never mind the fact that I was propelling a death box down the freeway at eighty miles per hour with my eyes closed. Never mind the lives of the countless strangers who were at heightened risk as I came swerving down Woodward Avenue. Never mind the precious life of the guy in the driver's seat—the one so full of promise and potential.

And never mind the guy who nearly killed him. He might even succeed as soon as tomorrow, when he does it all over again.

Never mind all of it. This morning I made it home.

Who knew when I arrived in this city that I'd learn so many ways to take away someone's life?

If that's not a recipe for sweet dreams, I don't know what is.

Track 5: THE MAGICAL MAN

Caleb's toothache would likely be the death of him.

Per his patient chart, two weeks before he arrived in the ER, Caleb had felt some discomfort in one of his molars. He had no dentist and no insurance, so he just hoped that the pain would go away on its own in a couple of days. It did not. Ten days went by, then he started to notice some swelling of the right side of his face. The next day, the swelling worsened, extending down into his neck. That night he woke suddenly with the feeling that his throat was closing up. He was right: the swelling had reached the tissue surrounding his vocal cords, threatening to suffocate him. An ambulance sped him to our doorstep, and within a couple of hours Caleb was in emergency surgery with one of my bosses, followed by the ICU, where his body's will to live would truly be tested.

It was just after midnight when I walked into Caleb's room and introduced myself to his unconscious body. High above his head hung several small bags—saline solution, insulin, electrolytes, antibiotics, vasopressors—all dripping slowly through a nest of tubing, each ultimately finding a path to his veins. The ventilator heaved away in the corner. I approached and began removing stained pieces of gauze from his neck.

To say his infection was aggressive was an understatement. Once it entered his neck, the bacteria had feasted—eating quickly through fat, fascia, and muscle. The natural barriers between neck structures had been destroyed, and the infection had found its way into major blood vessels and down into his chest. In the operating room, Caleb's neck had been sliced open from ear to ear and gutted like a sport fish. Most of the anatomy was unrecognizable, as everything had quickly decayed into a thick, foul-smelling soup.

Purulent fluid had been suctioned, unsalvageable tissue had been cut away, and flimsy hollow tubes of latex the caliber of garden hoses had been placed throughout the deep tissues of his neck to allow for the drainage of what our medical forefathers would have called "bad humors." We just call that shit pus.

His most optimistic chance for survival? Fifty percent.

Once all of the dressings were removed, I examined his neck. His incision was held together loosely by only a handful of sutures, the spaces between stitches occupied by wide silicone drains. Murky, brown, stinking fluid dripped from each—a sign that his infection continued to rage. I flushed several large syringes of saline into each drain to try to force the junk out of his neck and then wrapped his wound in clean gauze once again.

I cleaned up, turned to leave, and paused at the door. Something was strange about that room. I turned around and surveyed: monitors, vent, drugs, walls, lights, windows, drapes—everything seemed to check out. The patient, Caleb, had been a middle-aged Black man once but now looked barely human, as expected—when the neck has been splayed open and multiple tubes are stuffed into the mouth and nose of an unconscious face, it looks more like a Halloween mask. A swollen, rubbery imitation of life. And completely common for me to see on night rounds through the ICU. A tragically typical horror.

I must have been imagining things—there was nothing amiss in the stillness of Caleb's room. I was about to step out into the hallway when my eyes came to rest just below a folded visitors' chair propped against the window: five large clear plastic bags, each filled to the brim with clothing and other personal effects. The average patient showed up to the hospital with one, maybe two bags' worth of stuff, but *five*?

Then it hit me: this was *everything*. Caleb was homeless—a detail I'd missed in my cursory review of his history. All of his worldly possessions, all he had to his name—it all fit into five plastic bags, which he had likely forced the paramedics to pack into the ambulance with him.

The image gripped me. Caleb had no one by his side. He had no family or friends to contact, no home to which he would return, and no money save the handful of dollar bills tucked inside one of his plastic bags. I understood all of this in an instant. What kept me rooted to the floor of his doorway in that moment was the question of just when my mind had begun forming a new type of gut reaction, one both foreign and unnervingly casual:

Maybe he deserved it.

I drove home from the hospital several hours later, propelled into alertness by hunger. For some reason nearly all of my favorite restaurants were closed, so I ended up swinging into the drive-through of a fast-food joint, where I picked up a meal of delicious heart attack fuel. I was tearing into a grease-soaked cheeseburger on my living room sofa a few minutes later when my phone buzzed. It was my mom calling from the East Coast. And she wanted to video chat? Weird.

I took the call and found my screen filled with not only my mother's smiling face but also those of my two younger brothers. Weirder. They definitely didn't all live together at her house in Atlanta.

"Merry Christmas!" they proclaimed in unison.

Holy shit. I'd forgotten Christmas.

I exchanged pleasantries with my family for a few minutes

before begging off to go to bed. They didn't seem too upset that I'd neglected to send any presents this year, which only multiplied my guilt. Fucking residency, man.

As I lay cocooned in blankets moments later, my restless mind was consumed by the story of Christmas, the miraculous birth of Jesus, and all that followed. I felt a sudden need to get fresh air and popped my head out from underneath the covers. I stared up in confusion at the peeling paint on my ceiling.

Wait a second, I thought, *is Christmas some bullshit?*

Let's review.

So, Mary was a teenage virgin who'd been unexpectedly impregnated, not by the earthbound penis of the dude she was living with but *immaculately*, because God wanted to flex on humanity and show us that he could literally do *anything*. So her kid, Jesus, was born and everyone freaked the fuck out because nothing like that had ever happened before. A total miracle. At the very least, they should have followed up on this kid. Maybe spent some time postpartum asking Mary some gently probing questions. But nope—even though it seems like people loved to write shit down back then, there are no records of the kid's childhood or teenage years. Just his fantastical birth. Not weird at all. Fast-forward to Jesus as a grown man, preaching a gospel of inclusion, grace, and civility to anyone who will listen, all while he and his squad are *verrrrrry* heavily suggesting that he's the literal son of God. This assertion is supported from time to time by his performance of actual supernatural miracles all over the Middle East—turning water into wine (because a party was getting lame and his magical side recognized that people wanted to turn up; seriously, that's the story), routinely restoring sight to the blind with a few nice words and a touch from his hand (all you had to do was tell him you believed he was part deity and *bam*—twenty-twenty vision), etc. He gains a following, and those in power are none too pleased with the possibility of this guy becoming a major political force, so they kill him publicly and bury him in a cave. Three days later his supporters start circulating this wild story that they went to check on his body, but it had up and disappeared like David fucking Blaine. Later that day, Jesus showed up to hang with the squad a little bit and thank them for believing in him because, as they could see, he was definitely powerful beyond measure. He then moved on to heaven, where he is ostensibly watching over all of us at the right hand of his pops.

Jesus Christ—the only magical human in documented history. It sounded made up. Probably because it was.

That's okay, you know. These stories are clearly meant to be taken as allegories, not literal acts of magic.

Oh, really? You want to tell that to the West Indian Episcopalians who raised me to use white Jesus to justify our culture's self-hating colorism and use Bible verses to justify their desire to beat gay men to a pulp for fun? There's an entire world full of people who take the Bible's words literally. And even the reasonable ones who don't still believe in that final act of magic: the resurrection. That's the defining tenet of Christianity: blind belief in the magical man.

And for some reason, on that Christmas morning, that fact made me really fucking angry.

Because you felt lied to?

No, dude, it's not that simple. I mean, look at what that shit has led to. The magical man did magic tricks to corner us into believing in God. And for all of the flowery language he spewed about grace and mercy, in the end God is nothing but an all-powerful judge. It was God who gave us intelligent life, so our job is to prove to him/her/it that we were worth the fucking trouble. So we spend a lifetime judging ourselves. We form church communities so we can judge one another. Sunday after Sunday we shame one another into acting in accordance with the words some fucking lunatic on top of a mountain etched into stone. Those goddamn commandments. And what do we have to show for it? Not much more than the thin hope that we didn't fuck things up too much, because if we did, that omnipotent judge in the sky will sentence us to an eternity burning in hell.

We're supposed to be motivated through fear of damnation to give enough fucks about others, and dance on the razor's edge of "worthy" behavior. And in the end, it's all to save our own skin.

And you don't believe that's right. You haven't for a long time.

I mean, you were there when I was twelve. Back when I started asking questions about the magic. Of course, that led to asking questions about the politicians and amateur reporters who wrote the "Holy Bible." And finally it all led to my refusal to go to church again once I learned just how very much questions were unwelcome. So from then on I was—

On your own.

Yeah. As usual.

I mean, I knew deep down that there was something greater than me at work in this universe. I just had no framework through which I could understand it, let alone articulate it. All of the religion I'd known to that point was so vengeful and manipulative and full of convenient lapses in logic. So I wanted to start over. But . . . shit, you ever wonder what the construction of a new belief system—a whole new *religion*—sounds like when you're twelve years old? A whole lot of talking to yourself without much to show for it.

Searching for treasure without a map or a guide? You were always going to get lost. You should try taking it easy on yourself.

Not exactly my strongest suit, in case you haven't noticed.

We'll work on that. But I get it—you were a kid searching for meaning, looking for a sign that never came. Sure makes it hard to believe in whatever God is.

At the end of the day, "belief" was a bridge too far for me. I knew what I *wished* God was. Or rather, I knew what I wished God saw in me. I ~~needed to wanted to know~~ just hoped that my life and existence were more than a list of mistakes to be judged. I didn't want to be "loved" in the way that he loved his "son"—contingent upon the amount of abuse I could sustain up until the moment of my death. Love without any conditions. Love for the simple fact that I was here. Now *that* would have been magical.

But hope is flimsy. It won't sustain without evidence to bolster it. And I just could never see, or didn't understand, any signs that a higher power loved me.

Seriously? Let's just be objective: You're smart, talented, and healthy; despite the challenges in your way, you've somehow managed to continue achieving what so many others can't even dream of. Maybe it's luck. Or maybe that's what that elusive love looks like. I know you're in a shitty mood, but it feels like you're just being obstinately hopeless.

So you're saying that if I find myself balancing on a burning diving board one hundred feet above a pool filled with spikes and sharks, I should find comfort in the idea that "love" built the ladder I climbed?

All I've gained from those steps up is a longer, bloodier fall.

No, God doesn't love. Not me. Not any of us. I don't think it's within his capacity. It's probably just as I've always been taught—God is there to watch, to judge, to siphon us into the fire when we die. Because there are no saints among us. We've all been cruel, we've all been selfish, we've all brought pain. We've all sinned. And judges rule based on what we've done. Not how sorry we are for having done it. So odds are, we're all destined to burn.

You asked me earlier if I pray. My initial answer was "Fuck no. What's the point?" I don't think that's true anymore.

Lately I've been praying that we've all gotten it wrong. And I feel that I may be onto something, because these days prayers have become screams into an echoless abyss. They're shots of blind hope that when it's all over for me, for Caleb, for any one of us . . . the only thing that awaits us is darkness.

You asked me what I believe in. This is it: nothingness.

That's the only true freedom I can imagine. No place for judgment to exist, and so nothing to fear. No God lying in wait. The lights just go out. A simple end.

That simplifies life quite a bit, doesn't it? Whether I do good or bring suffering, whether I grieve a loss or keep rounding, none of it fucking matters.

That's got to be why I don't feel any of the deaths I've witnessed. There's nothing mystical about the end of a life. It's not some grand tragedy. Death is a sequence of mechanical failures, nothing more and nothing less. A machine simply breaks down and stops. Usually it makes a handful of people sad for a short time, then they move on with their lives because there's shit to do. Until their machines fail. Life goes on till it doesn't. What we do on the way doesn't change where we end up.

Nothing matters.

I know this is the part where you, my ever-encouraging shoulder angel, tell me I'm wrong. That there's love and meaning in this life. That my childish wish that God could be those things could be true if only I'd let the possibility in.

Well, prove it, motherfucker. I'll wait.

And when you're ready, why don't you go ahead and explain it to the man whose life fits into five fucking shopping bags. Explain to him that it wasn't bad luck or bad choices or evil deeds that got him there.

Tell him it was love.

Go ahead. I fucking dare you.

On December 26 I arrived at the hospital to find that Caleb's name was no longer on my patient list. A series of mechanical failures. A new critically ill body had already replaced him in the ICU. His bags were likely in a dumpster outside.

I loosed a parting prayer into the void for Caleb—the simple hope that, like me, he'd relinquished all attachments to religion and meaning, any fantasies of something more.

Because in this harsh, unforgiving world we were given . . . tethered to these fragile, desperate lives we've created . . .

In the face of death . . .

Believing in something is so much more painful than believing in nothing at all.

Next patient.

Track 6: ELEVATORS

For the first twenty-one years of my life, I drank exactly zero sips of alcohol.

It wasn't because I resided on a moral high ground or because I held a firm belief that minors should always abide by society's laws. The simple reason was that, compared with my peers, I felt I had more to lose if I lost control of myself. Chalk it up to a combination of my low-level paranoid neuroses and the recognition of what my Blackness meant in a sea of white high school students of privilege. Even then I knew that my SPF 50–drenched friends[5] would walk through life in this country on a smoothly paved road, while I'd walk beside them on a tightrope trying desperately not to fall with each step.

America didn't love me enough to forgive my mistakes.

So tipsy tightroping just didn't make much sense to me.

For most of college, I took on the role of Sober Party Bro-Mom: I was the dude who was just as uninhibited and partied just as hard as his drunk friends but made sure that everyone made it back to the dorms at the end of the evening's shenanigans. Some nights I'd roll a sleeping friend onto his stomach and position a trash bin near his head, as he had a tendency to puke in his sleep. Other nights I'd find my roommate passed out, pantsless, on the floor of our bathroom and I'd gently drape a towel over his butt because

a. I knew that the combined unforgiving chill of both linoleum on his genitals and bare ass cheeks in the breeze would prove too much to bear come morning; and

b. dignity.

Although I was never jealous of anyone's good time under the influence, I increasingly coveted their freedom. Black history in

---

5. I hold firm to the conviction that the only thing white people fear—like, the *only* thing they worry might destroy them—is the fucking sun. The one thing that makes life possible on this Earth, and it burns their skin off even when it's cloudy. The irony makes me giggle my ass off.

America had led me to believe that success required me to curtail my baser impulses lest I end up dead or in jail, but I was starting to feel a nagging rebellious itch. Why couldn't I do dumb shit from time to time and still manage to graduate from college? White people did it all the time, right? So for my twenty-first birthday, since I'd no longer be breaking any laws by getting boozed up, we threw a "Let's Get Tony Hammered for the First Time in History" party at a local bar. I hung up my Bro-Mom cape and finally threw all caution to the wind.

My very first alcoholic beverage slid across the bar courtesy of my roommate (the one whom I'd *finally* taught to do his own laundry): a Bombay Sapphire gin and tonic. It was so delicious and so motherfucking *refreshing* that I convinced myself that it had to, somehow, be good for my health. I could almost taste the secret vitamins giving me strength and vitality with each sip.

I had three more, just to start my night off.

Things got weird, loud, and more than a little bit dizzy.

I woke up the next morning on my bedroom floor to a surprising realization: the whole world had shown up to get me drunk the night before, but I'd still been the one to get myself home safely. I'd stumbled through streets and dorm corridors, vomited somewhere along the way, somehow sprained my ankle, and bruised an entire side of my head when I'd fallen into my bed and missed. None of my friends had taken the time to be *my* Bro-Mom. Not a got-damn one of them.

So one of two conclusions had to be true: either my friends were the worst people of all time, or for the last three years I had been a complete and utter chump for helping them through the moments they wouldn't remember.

As I peeled my face off my carpet and teased a stray blond hair (of uncertain origin) from between my teeth, I arrived at the verdict: I had been the owner of a shitty duplex on 21 Chump Street, located in the historic East Chumpington Lake neighborhood of downtown Chump City.

Drunk friends hadn't been there for me, so I wouldn't be there for them. Kindness and effort and care need to go both ways, you sloppy motherfuckers.

Meanwhile, ten years later, somewhere in America's heartland . . .

"Guys, I'm sorry but I have to interrupt for, like, three seconds."

Hae Won's head emerged slowly from the neck of his plaid field coat like a baby-faced tortoise. Our band of merry surgical residents craned our necks over the sticky bar of Ye Olde Saloon (the dive-iest of dive bars in the Detroit suburbs) to hear Hae Won's forthcoming sage words. He had been pensive for the last fifteen minutes.

"Ye Olde . . ." he said, as if this alone were a thesis statement. "*Yeeeeee Olde!*"

Beside me, Z smirked and flipped her glossy hair out of her face. "This is gonna be amazing," she muttered to herself.

Hae Won continued, eyes wide, "'Ye' is totally not a thing. Well, it is a thing. Everything is a thing. But we say 'ye' only because there used to be an old letter that represented the 'th' sound, and that shit looked like a Y. So we *should* be saying 'the olde,' but we just like the way that *yeeeeeeee* feels!"

"*Yat* shit is crazy!" exclaimed Z. Nailed it.

"High thoughts with Hae Won, everyone. Be sure to tip your waitress," I said, preparing to take another sip of domestic beer.

"Man, these aren't high thoughts. These are *real* thoughts!" pleaded Hae Won.

I couldn't help but chuckle. Hae Won was most definitely high. He had a tendency to wax pedantic when he had marijuana in his system, and he'd had a couple of hits in the bar's parking lot.

Z's ebullience could not be contained. She hooted and raised her arm for a high five. "These may, in fact, be the realest thoughts of all time!" Her palm met ye olde palm of Hae Won just centimeters from my face.

"Okay, so can I please continue my story? It. Is. Whit. Ney. Sto. Ry. Time!" Whitney exclaimed, clapping her hands excitedly with each syllable. At the commanding height of six foot one, Whitney towered over those of us seated at the bar.

"So we meet in the call room last week and we are trying desperately to have sex," continued Whitney, "and it's all knees and elbows. I literally cannot find a spot where I'm not bumping into something, because I'm the tallest woman on earth and we are on a twin mattress on the bottom of a fucking bunk bed!"

"Not only that," I added, "but ain't no lumbar support in those beds. You're not a teenager, damn it. You've got to be thinking long term about lower-back problems!"

Z stole a knowing glance at me over her glass as she took a swig of vodka.

"EXACTLY!" Whitney shouted, her midwestern lilt now in full swing. "So I told him, 'Listen, I'm a *lady*. I don't have sex on bunk beds like a desperate college kid. You need to figure out a solution.' So he texts me when we're both on call last night and tells me he's got something special planned. I show up to the call room and the top bunk is fucking *gone*."

I nearly spit out my beer. "YESSSSSSSS!"

"But . . . how?" whispered Hae Won into the marijuana-tainted ether.

"This dude called maintenance and had them remove the top bunk," Whitney replied, raising her mug of Blue Moon to the sky. "Because I'm apparently so good in the sack that you need to hire an interior decorator in a hospital just to have another CHANCE. WITH. THIS. Annnnnnd I thank you."

She curtsied, and we slow-clapped in admiration.

"Know what?" Z stood up and, after some light swaying, managed to land a hand on Whitney's shoulder. "Fuck George Washington. Fuck Abraham Lincoln. And fuck the fucking Statue of Liberty. YOU ARE THE TRUE AMERICAN PATRIOT!"

"Protecting us from fucked-up-ass furniture, foreign and domestic," added Hae Won.

I ordered a round of shots. Whiskey. Each young surgeon raised a glass of liquid amnesia to the sky.

"To Whitney," I declared, "the actual American dream. May you continue to topple the patriarchy one bunk bed smash at a time."

We were the future lifesavers of America, each of us training in a different surgical specialty—from brain stuff all the way south, down to butt stuff. We were brilliant, dedicated, and talented. And in the precious moments that we owned outside of work, all of our social activities centered around, or were adorned by, liquor, drugs, and sex. Self-preservation by way of self-medication. We were all aware that we were doing it—we were smart kids, after all. The reality was that each of us walked the hospital corridors each day with varying degrees of pain, sadness, insecurity, and desperation bubbling just beneath our skin. All of the things we'd been taught a surgeon is *not* supposed to be and, simultaneously, all of the things that the job encouraged and emboldened. So we played mind games with ourselves, stretching our neurons within millimeters of their lives to convince ourselves that we were okay—that we were stronger and smarter than our frivolous, obstructive emotions. But that's a dangerous game. Those intrusive reminders of your vulnerability don't just go away. They beg to be recognized, answered, navigated, and fucking *dealt with*. The problem is, when you can feel the fragility of the frayed connections inside your own head, tugging at them for clarity with shit like self-interrogation, meaningful conversations, or <gasp> *therapy* seems like a surefire way to snap them apart irreparably. And if that happened, if we were crushed under the weight of our pent-up (completely normal and reasonable, btw) human feelings, how could we go on? More important, how could we continue doing our jobs?

We couldn't. And that wasn't an option.

So we'd drink. And we'd smoke. And we'd dampen the sheets of the call rooms' (former) bunk beds. Because it was fun. And because at a certain point each night, we'd find comfort in trapping our emotions in a vice-fueled fog where they couldn't threaten to hurt us again until morning. It was just easier that way. And we were desperate for at least one part of our lives to be easy.

One night, Z and I attended a party hosted by some older residents with whom we weren't very familiar. We pregamed at her house with several cups of a college-style beverage known as a Pink Panty Dropper—a rose-tinted concoction of cheap vodka, even cheaper beer, and a can of frozen pink lemonade mix. True to its name, the power of the PPD bulldozed inhibitions and supercharged libidos, and we found ourselves sloppily making out on a couch in a strange house, surrounded by gawking strangers and coworkers. After far too long, we realized our folly and, like classy adults, relocated to the guest bathroom, where we had sloppy sex all over their bathroom fixtures, including a sink that we managed to break clean off the wall. Now, on the one hand: crisp high five for epic boot knocking? On the other hand: ABSOLUTELY NOT COOL. To anyone in their right, sober mind this was a completely unacceptable, totally obnoxious antic to pull as a guest in someone's house. I mean, have crazy bathroom sex in your own home all you want, but don't wipe sweaty balls and butt cheeks on the same porcelain where a stranger rests his toothbrush, and then snap it off the goddamn wall. Jesus.

The hosts were gracious enough to our faces, refusing to let us pay for the repair and assuring us that it was no big deal. But in the sober light of the next morning, as I woke up choking on Z's silky mane of auburn hair, I knew that our behavior was actually a very large deal. We were the drunken assholes who'd managed to fuck a sink off a wall in a stranger's house. My mother had to have raised me better than that.

Perhaps, I thought, it was time to take a break from casual binge drinking.

A few weeks later a nondoctor buddy, Wally, threw himself a birthday party at a bar in downtown Detroit, and I volunteered to be <gasp> *the designated driver* for a few friends in my neighborhood. Amazingly enough, I wasn't lamenting a night without booze. The promise of a night out on the town with a bunch of people who had nothing to do with the hospital had put some canned heat in my heels[6] and I was ready to responsibly rage in fancy attire. Now, secondary to poverty, I had not gone shopping

---

6. What's that, you say? This is the first Jamiroquai reference you've heard outside of *Napoleon Dynamite* in twenty-plus years? Thank you, and you're welcome.

for new clothes in several years. As a result, I'd become a master of what I call *squinty chic*: an outfit that looks super hip and classy, as long as you don't look too close and you kind of squint your eyes. My "fancy" jeans had a minor two-centimeter hole in the crotch, so I had to be on the lookout for any requests that I assume spread-eagle positions; I polished my one pair of brown dress shoes with an alcohol swab (probably not great for the faux leather) and put on fresh socks to mask the odor that wafted from their soles; and I donned my favorite (read: only) blazer over a freshly ironed button-down shirt so as to avoid bringing attention to the inevitable pit-sweat stains. From six feet away, I would look and smell like a supermodel. There would be nothing but winning for old Chin-Quee on this brisk Detroit night.

I did end up inviting two doctor friends to the party, neither of whom worked at my hospital, so I was able to maintain an appropriate gulf of emotional separation from my job. Sawyer and Katya, both surgery residents, had been wound pretty tightly at work lately, so when I extended the invitation, they jumped at the opportunity to put on fancy clothes and cut loose for a few precious hours. I'd met Katya a year earlier at a Halloween party. She'd come as a high school frog dissection gone wrong, with full-body green makeup, huge glassy dead eyeballs superimposed on her own, abdominal skin pulled back and tacked to her sides, and belly anatomy expertly reproduced in gory detail. She'd done it all by herself with nothing but paints, a mirror, and a glass of wine. She was an artist masquerading as a surgeon, just like me. We understood each other instantly.

She planned to meet us at the venue, while Sawyer hopped into the back seat of my carpool with a flask of whiskey in hand. Skilled

in the fine Canadian arts of wilderness survival, bacon preparation, and Olympic-level Eskimo ear pulling,[7] Sawyer always seemed
more lumberjill than surgeon—a characteristic that made us fast
friends. I would have deemed the car flask a trashy move had it not
been for the proud Canadian flag emblazoned on its side. Seeing as
I believe in the inherent adorableness of all Canadians (nearly as
much as I believe in sweeping cultural generalizations), I was compelled to allow it. I hit the gas and chauffeured a gaggle of tipsy
ladies into the night.

The birthday festivities were held in a bar that occupied the top
floor of the Whitney, one of the oldest mansions in Detroit. Initially built and occupied at the turn of the twentieth century by
lumber baron David Whitney, every inch of the place dripped with
opulence. Every wall of the foyer was adorned with sculpted
sconces, mirrors in gilt frames, and more fireplaces per square foot
than reason could account for. The foyer ended in a grand carpeted staircase, the first landing of which served as a viewing area
for two Tiffany glass windows.[8] The best part was that everything
smelled like really fancy wood—the floors, the table decorations,
even the tuxedoed servers trailed a certain *eau de bois* behind
them as they walked by.

True to form, my armpits couldn't help but water in the rar-
efied air of old lumber wealth. The blazer was a good choice.

The Ghostbar, so named due to the undead spirits of the Whitney family that were said to still walk the halls of the house, was

---

7. An actual sport. Look it up and then definitely try it at home with your friends and loved ones.
You won't be sorry.
8. With some quick research, I learned that Tiffany glass windows are essentially your favorite
stained-glass window's favorite stained-glass window. The Whitney is home to several of these, their
collective worth likely exceeding the worth of one hundred Tonys in one hundred lifetimes.

bubbling with smartly dressed partygoers. Softly lit lamps hung low from the ornate vaulted ceiling, casting unnatural shadows on the mahogany furnishings and creating an ambience of quiet, eerie decadence. As if in response, the guests conversed in hushed murmurs as their high heels and boat shoes shuffled silently across the carpet. And yes, that's right, the entire bar floor was covered with an ancient luxury carpet. It was a bold move on the part of old man Whitney, one that demanded his guests never spill a drop of liquor on the floor, lest they incur the wrath of the many house ghosts.

I turned to Sawyer. "They have shit like this in Canada?"

Sawyer raised a single eyebrow as she took in the scene. "I'm not blown away. Céline Dion has like six of these." She tucked her hair behind her ear as she leaned in close and whispered, "Have you ever sung 'My Heart Will Go On' barefoot on a moose-hide rug?"

"Have you?" I asked.

She winked at me. "That's Canadian luxury, my friend. Let's go see if this place is too fancy to put whiskey in a cup for me."

My friends are weirdos.

We took up residence at the bar, and I ordered a gin and tonic from the elderly bartender, the only other Black face in the room. My eyes swept the crowd. The ladies looked alluring and mysterious in the bar's mood lighting—a perfect venue in which to babysit my single drink and engage in the search for a future heartbreak. A commotion at the far end of the bar caught my attention as a handful of men jockeyed for the attention of one woman. *Jackpot, baby.* I summoned my legendary swagger to the surface as I leaned over the bar for a better look. A lithe, dark-haired woman held court in a sheer, thigh-length black cocktail dress. She had the boys eating out of the palm of her hand—with each gesture and every word, they erupted in laughter and tried to inch just a bit closer. She turned to grab a sip of her martini, caught my eye, and shattered the decorum of the room as she screamed, "YESSSSSS, CHIN-QUEE! WHAT IT DO?!"

Classic Katya. Even in scrubs, her beauty would regularly strike men dumb. Seeing her in that low-cut, nearly see-through dress, those boys didn't stand a chance. And my homegirl Katya was eating it up. She waved me over.

I parted the sea of men and joined her. "Why do you do this to these poor boys, K? They really shouldn't be drooling on this expensive-ass carpet."

She threw her head back and let out a husky laugh. I was always surprised by how deep her voice was. "Gimme a break, homie. Sometimes a girl just needs to feel sexy, you know?" She threw back the remaining martini and exhaled slowly as it burned down her throat. "Besides, it's not my fault that these boys don't know how to handle any of *this*." She swung her hips in a sultry arc, all while eyeing a bespectacled suitor to her right. I could see the beads of sweat on his forehead as he sipped his beer anxiously. Poor bastard.

She raised a triumphant eyebrow at me and reached for her glass, which had already been cleared by the bartender. "Oh, what the fuck," she hissed. "Fuck that efficient-ass motherfucker."

"Easy there, champ, I got you." I bought her a fresh martini, and she raised the glass in a salute to my generosity before downing a generous gulp. I left her to her man harem and continued my stroll about the room.

An hour floated by, and the once politely murmuring voices had crescendoed into a raucous, drunken din. A sweet haze of cigar smoke hung just overhead, and the hands of the geriatric bartender were a blur as he whipped together Prohibition-era drinks. I avoided venomous looks from a couple of girls I'd never called back after one date and did my best to feign interest in the words of the voluptuous redhead in front of me. She was a teacher at Pure Barre, which sounded like a workout class for white women of privilege wherein they do ballet stretches for an hour until they kind of sweat a little. And *OMG, it had totally changed her life.* Sigh. I was calculating the annoyance-to-benefit ratio of giving this woman a tour of my bedroom that night when a new commotion broke out.

Several partygoers huddled in a circle, staring at something just below eye level. Wally emerged from the crowd and beckoned me over.

"I think you should take care of this, buddy," he said, pointing toward the crowd. I pushed my way through to find Sawyer bent over a barstool, heaving vomit all over a carpet that was likely worth more than my entire life. The crowd looked on in disgust, inching away with each wretch to protect their shoes.

Oh, Canada. Not great.

I knelt down and swept a shock of blond hair behind her ear. She looked up at me, eyes glazed and bloodshot but still as playful as ever.

"How do I look?" she croaked.

"Well, you're ass over head on a barstool, and I'm pretty sure you have old puke bacon in your hair," I replied. "So overall, I'd say pretty good."

"That's a relief." She wiped her mouth with the back of her hand. "I think I broke their carpet."

I looked down at the venerable old carpet, now smothered in partially digested, whiskey-soaked dinner. I squinted at what appeared to be three intact pieces of popcorn in the mess. How was that even possible?

"I think it'll be fine. They were planning on redecorating anyway."

"Really?"

"No, not really. Not at all," I looked up at the onlookers, squirming in their suits and dresses. Not even an offer of a paper towel from any of them.

"So what do you say?" I patted her gently on the back. "Home?"

She nodded. "Home."

I propped her up against me and we left the bar, carefully descending the stairs to the lobby. Gathering the remainder of my friends to leave immediately in my car would have proved as easy as herding a bunch of wet, drunk cats, so I decided to call a taxi to bring Sawyer home. We waited on the sidewalk outside the mansion. Sawyer stood in the frigid night air without a shiver, staring up at the sky, swaying slowly from side to side.

"Tony." She let out a long, pained sigh. "I miss dick."

"What's that, now?"

"Penis, Chin-Quee! I miss all of them. All of the penises. I just . . . I want them near me. I want them near my face . . . and in my body holes . . . and I want . . . I miss the men . . . who are attached to them." Her eyes locked on mine with a desperate intensity. This had been eating at her for ages. I remained silent.

"And Erin is, like, super great," she continued. "She's a really good girlfriend, and she's super patient, and she's really . . . She's my best friend at work and outside of work. But I think she knows. I mean, I told her at the start that I'd never done the girl dating thing before, and she said not to worry because she's only ever done the girl dating thing so she could show me how it goes . . . so

I did it, and I'm doing it, and I don't . . . Like, what's wrong with me that I can't just love this person who loves me so fucking much? I just . . . She . . . she doesn't have enough penis."

I nodded. "Yeah, I'd imagine it's hard for her to find enough . . . penis."

She dropped her head to her chest and let out another long sigh.

"So why don't you just tell her how you feel?"

She shook her head and laid it to rest on my shoulder.

"Because." Her voice was muffled against my jacket. "I don't know how to be more lonely than this."

I put an arm around her as she fell into silence. Her shoulders shuddered as she began to cry. The taxi arrived a moment later. I shuffled my feet to help Sawyer to the door of the car and stepped on something slippery. I looked down and found that she hadn't been crying at all. My shoes and jeans were streaked with fresh vomit, steaming in the night air. That sneaky fucking Canadian.

She looked up at me. "I think I broke your shoes."

I smiled and helped her into the back seat. "Just make sure you keep the window rolled down."

The cabdriver shouted out the passenger-side window at me, "Hey, man, is she okay?"

"Oh yeah, bro, she's great!" His eyes caught a glimpse of my pants. I held a hand up just as he was opening his mouth in protest. "Don't worry, my friend," I said. "This mess is all mine. I am very, very drunk."

He looked at me skeptically.

I continued, "You're lucky it's not me in the back seat. She'll be awesome."

Maybe.

The cab sped off into the night, and I hustled back into the mansion in search of a restroom.

When I emerged from the bathroom, my pants still damp from a rapid puke scrub, I found Wally hustling down the staircase. Three strands of his carefully coiffed hair had fallen onto his forehead, and his cherubic cheeks were flushed. He approached with the comically deliberate stride of a man looking to maintain order in spite of his total drunkenness.

"Hey, buddy, I was just looking for you!"

"Hey, man," I said sheepishly, "I'm so sorry about Sawyer up there. I'd offer to pay for the carpet but . . . I gotta be honest with you, this is my best pair of jeans. It's got fresh vomit residue and a hole in the crotch so big I can feel every gust of wind in my fucking loins. And I'm probably gonna wear them again tomorrow."

Wally smiled. "Dude, seriously, don't worry about it. You're not the one who puked, and that carpet has definitely seen worse."

"Yeah, you're probably right. So . . . what's up, man?"

Wally summoned a deep breath and let it out slowly. "Okay. So, the elevator isn't working. We think it might be stuck between floors. Someone saw your doctor friend waiting on it a few minutes ago, and now nobody can find her."

Katya. Shit.

The dial above the elevator door next to the staircase indicated that the car was stuck between the second and third floors. I whipped out my phone and called her—straight to voice mail. I sent a quick barrage of texts, all variations on "Hey, is your ass trapped in a rickety mansion elevator that is unlikely to be up to code?" Nary a three-dot bubble in response. This was definitely not great.

Wally and I sprinted up to the third-floor landing. A warm glow peeked through the lower half of the slim gap between the closed elevator doors. I pounded on the doors as I yelled Katya's name—no answer. I turned to Wally.

"Are there emergency elevator guys that we can call?" I asked.

"I already asked someone in maintenance to check. Apparently the earliest anyone can get here is six a.m."

I started to feel panic rise in my throat. What had happened to make that elevator stop? And why the hell wasn't she *answering*? "Who else can we call? The fire department?"

I could see Wally wade through a fog of drunkenness to consider this. "Well, the elevator doesn't seem to be on fire," he began, "but they do get called to get cats out of trees in the movies. Was Keanu Reeves a fireman in *Speed*?"

"Where you going with this, big guy?"

"*Speed*, man! Keanu Reeves saved a whole bunch of people from an elevator in the first scene, right? Wasn't he some sort of badass fireman?"

I did not have time for Wally's failures at nineties movie trivia. "He was on a fucking SWAT team, dude. He was doing badass elevator shit because Dennis Hopper rigged the fucking thing to a bomb." I sighed and rested my head against the elevator door. "If there's anyone who'd know what to do right now, it would be motherfucking Keanu Reeves."

I closed my eyes and tried to regain my composure. My sarcasm wasn't helping. It wasn't Wally's fault that he was bad at drunken problem-solving. And it certainly wasn't Keanu Reeves's fault. He's a fucking international treasure. He's a man of action, rugged good looks, and kung fu skills. And if he were here he'd . . .

My head jolted back up. The gap between the elevator doors was just large enough for the tips of my fingers to find a grip. I had no idea how heavy the doors might be, but we were clearly out of options. I found purchase for all ten of my fingers, bent my knees, took in a deep breath, and pulled. Hard. *One second . . . two seconds . . .* Nothing. *This was a dumb idea . . . three seconds . . . four seconds . . .* Still nothing. At this point I was embarrassing myself in front of the rapidly growing crowd of spectators. *Five seconds . . .* A sudden plaintive, metallic groan escaped from somewhere inside the elevator shaft. The gap widened by a couple of centimeters. *Keep pushing . . . six seconds . . . seven seconds . . .* The gap widened farther; my shoulder muscles burned in protest. I slipped my palms between the doors and gripped them on the inside. I took another deep breath and heaved. The two doors shot out to either side.

Can we just take a moment to acknowledge that you winning against an elevator door is objectively awesome? If I had friends to talk to, they'd never hear the end of it.

Honestly, I don't think I could do it again. It was definitely a combination of mother-lifting-a-bus-off-her-baby adrenaline strength and an elevator that was over a century old. Nevertheless, worthy of *Matrix*-era Keanu Reeves comparisons?

I'll allow it.

Fuck yeah.

Moving on.

The roof of the elevator car hung in the dark shaft at waist level. I knelt down, peered into the car, and saw Katya sprawled motionless on the floor, miniskirt hiked up above her waist, the contents of her handbag scattered about her head. I swung my legs over the ledge and hopped down into the stalled car. The elevator gave an unnerving bounce as I hit the floor. Somewhere in the shaft above me metal squealed on metal. Shit. Fuck elevators. They really never should have invented these things in the first place.

I quickly went to my knees just above Katya's head, bent down to her face, and listened. Short, gurgling breaths escaped her mouth every few seconds. Her lips weren't blue yet, but she wouldn't hang on like this for too long. As I listened, I pressed two fingers into the side of her upper neck and found a slow, regular pulse. Good. We like pulses. With my left hand I pulled out my cell phone and flipped on the flashlight function, and with my right I cranked her mouth open with my thumb and index finger. Her mouth was clear, as far as I could see. I straightened her onto her back, tilted her head back, and thrust her jaw forward with both hands. The gurgling ceased almost immediately, replaced by clear, soft breaths, but she still wasn't breathing *often* enough. Seven or eight times a minute, by my quick calculation.

She was limp as a rag doll. I shouted her name into her ear and slapped her chest a few times. Nothing. I balled my hand into a fist and dug the knuckle of my middle finger into the middle of her rib cage with the weight of my upper body. This is a technique called a sternal rub: a type of noxious stimulus, our fancy term for "something so fucking immediately painful it should wake your ass up." She didn't budge.

Come on, Katya.

I looked up and saw Wally kneeling at the elevator door one floor up. "Wally, do me a favor," I shouted. "Call 911 and tell them what's going on. But first, check that bunch of people behind you and find the two dudes with the least amount of drunkenness and largest amount of upper body strength. I need to talk to them."

I looked over at the buttons next to the elevator door. Every floor's button was lit, and the emergency stop switch had been pulled. I went to the panel and tried pushing the switch back in. Nothing, just a soft bounce of the elevator car and the distant groan of metal above us. *Don't major in elevator sciences*, they said. *That degree will never pay off*, they said. If I died in that hanging metal box, I was going to dedicate my tombstone to those practical-ass, hating-ass haters.

Two well-barbered, slightly flushed faces appeared above me in the doorway.

"Hey, boys," I shouted. "She's in bad shape, and I don't really know how safe this elevator is, so we're gonna lift her out of here. Each of you grab an arm with one hand and put your other hand behind her head. Do *not* let her head hit anything hard. Ready?"

Blank stares all around.

Fuck it. That would have to be good enough.

I bent down, scooped my arms underneath Katya's torso, and stood up quickly. There was another shriek of the antique metal-work above me. I bent my knees and heaved her limp body up to my shoulder. The boys above had gotten down onto their bellies and slid their upper bodies into the elevator car. Each grabbed a limp arm and cradled the back of her head and neck. On my count, I pushed as they pulled, and Katya disappeared onto the landing. I hoisted my body up and out onto solid ground. I turned around and managed a last glance at the bouncing elevator car, its open face wheezing a last mirthless laugh.

Stairs from now on. Definitely stairs.

With Wally clearing the way ahead of us, we swept through the crowd and into a vacant sitting room. Once we got Katya situated safely on a couch, I sat next to her head and thrust her jaw forward again. She continued to breathe, albeit infuriatingly infrequently. I'd seen patients like this in the emergency room. Unless Katya had a drug problem that I didn't know about, this was alcohol poison-ing. Booze can be very sneaky inside the human body: you can feel pleasantly tipsy until well after your last drink and then, all of a sudden, the sauce will cause sudden power outages within vital organs like the brain. Looking down at her face, tranquil in the repose of a light coma, I replayed every moment I'd spent with Katya that night. She had to have been wasted before she'd even shown up to the party. *How had I missed it?*

A moment later, a team of paramedics bounded into the room. I told them an abridged version of the night's adventure as they scurried around my friend performing the well-rehearsed dance of emergency stabilization. In seconds, she was secured to a stretcher with an oxygen mask over her face and a monitor at her feet that chirped out her vital signs. I told the paramedics that I'd hold on to her belongings and bring them over to her at the hospital after I dropped off the remainder of my carpool. Which hospital would they be headed to?

County.

As in Katya's place of work, where she was scheduled to begin a shift in a few hours.

I pulled aside the lead paramedic and asked quietly if there was any way they could make sure she was placed in a secluded area of the ER. She was an employee, and any discretion they could afford her would be greatly appreciated.

He'd see what they could do. The team rolled Katya quickly out the door toward the main staircase.

I collected the remainder of my drunk friends from the bar and drove them back to the suburbs. I texted one of Katya's friends, an emergency room resident at County, asking if, on the off chance she was working, she could check on Katya and bring her a set of scrubs to change into for her morning shift. She was and she could. Finally, a bit of overdue luck.

When I got to the hospital, I saw that the paramedics had done well: Katya was in the secluded corner of the ER traditionally reserved for the psychiatrically unstable, and she was the only patient. IV fluid ran dutifully into her veins as she lay unresponsive. I smiled at the set of scrubs folded at the foot of the bed, and I placed her wallet, keys, and cell phone on top.

The clock on the wall was ticking toward 3:00 a.m. I dropped into a chair, overcome with exhaustion. It was far past my bedtime, and soreness was creeping quickly into my elevator-domination shoulder muscles. Katya's words from earlier in the night found their way back to my mind as my eyelids got heavy. She had come out that night looking to feel something; to find a little piece of her that she'd misplaced somewhere along the way. She might have succeeded only in glimpsing a shadow of it for a few moments, long enough to smell its passing, familiar scent before she'd lost all time. Perhaps she'd remember those moments when she woke. Or maybe she'd only know the paralyzing fear of losing everything as she recognized the pattern of the curtains and the shade of the linoleum underfoot.

I stood and stretched, staving off the threat of sleep. There was nothing more I could do. I made my way back to my car, cranked the music, and cracked the window to ensure an invigorating, icy breeze. As I threw the car into gear, I couldn't shake the feeling that I might actually have done *too* much.

My phone rang just after noon, waking me from the last throes of a fitful sleep.

"Hey, dude." Katya's husky voice was music to my ears.

"Morning, sunshine," I replied as I wiped the sleep out of my eyes. "Did you make it to rounds?"

"Yeah. I was only fifteen minutes late, actually." She paused. "So . . . what happened last night?"

I recounted the night's exploits, sparing no detail as I helped reconstruct her memories. She listened silently, occasionally asking questions and filling in the details that she could recall. As it turned out, she'd drunk two bottles of wine by herself before showing up to the party. She'd worn it well—no one was the wiser as she'd doubled down on martinis at the Ghostbar.

There was a long silence after I'd finished.

"Why didn't you tell the ambulance guys to take me to a different hospital?"

"Honestly, I didn't know you could do that," I said.

She let out a long sigh. "Yeah, Tony, you can do that."

This was not going well. "Listen, K, I'm really sorry. I did everything I could to—"

"I mean, why did you even call the ambulance in the first place?" Her voice was rising. "You could have just brought me home and put me to bed and everything would have probably been fine. I mean, all morning I was walking around wondering if anyone from my program had seen me in the ER. I keep waiting for my program director to call me into his office to fire me. I mean, fucking Christ, dude, this is my *life*!"

I took in a long breath. "Katya, you've got to trust me and know that I didn't have a choice. I found you unresponsive on the floor of an elevator. I had no idea how long you'd been there, no idea why you were unconscious, no idea if you had vomit in your lungs, no idea if you'd hit your head on something. Slinging you over my shoulder and bringing you to your apartment was not an option."

Silence on the other end of the line.

"Look," I continued, "I'm sorry you ended up at County. I really am. I did everything I could to make sure that nobody ran into you while you were all fucked up. The odds are that the only thing your program director will know is that you were late this morning. Believe me, I feel you—this is mortifying. But I'm just relieved that you're okay."

More silence. This time I sat in it with her, for nearly a minute.

"So, I spoke with Kim this morning," she said finally, "and she said that she saw you buying me a bunch of drinks last night." She paused, then in a halting whisper, added, "She said she saw you getting really handsy and trying to kiss me."

Kim is a good friend of Katya's whom I'd known in passing for the last year. She had introduced me to a nondoctor woman whom I'd dated and subsequently broken up with in spectacular fashion. Since then, I'd been pretty much dead to her. I'd dodged several daggers from her eyes the night before as I worked the room.

Additionally, *fuck Kim*. What kind of person would sow a seed like this in her friend's mind, based not on what she saw but on what she thinks I'm capable of?

Okay, don't bite my head off, but . . . even though she was factually wrong—you didn't know Katya was drunk when you bought her the one drink, and you made no moves to take advantage of her physically or sexually—is it possible that there might be a lesson to be learned from how Kim perceived you?

Are you fucking kidding me right now?

Just hear me out. You remember yourself as the reluctant hero of this story, and I get that—it was traumatic, and you need a way to process it that lets you look yourself in the face in the morning, so you've created a version that suits you. It's a thing you do with quite a bit of frequency, actually. But you've got to think beyond your conscious intent and interrogate the misogyny that laces your thoughts and actions so casually that it's invisible to you.

I was listening to your words. And I know your moves at a bar. You were patrolling for girls with a cocktail in your hand all night. You're a close talker when it's loud. And you definitely touch people as you talk to them. Your descriptors for Katya when you saw her tonight? About her dress and her body? You might have been quiet about it, but you were lusting after her just as much as the crowd of dudes who were hounding her. You telling me that if she had given you any semblance of a green light you wouldn't have—

I'm sorry—first of all, fuck you. You telling me it's fine to be accused of some shit I didn't do because of, what, unspoken intentions I didn't even know I was having?

It's just a different perspective. And given the numbers that I know *you know—at least eight out of every ten women has experienced some form of sexual harassment or assault—it's likely a very prevalent* female *perspective on your "harmlessness." A perspective that Kim and Katya walk around with every single day. And one that you're free to ignore because you're a fucking* dude.

Look, I know it sucks not to get the pat on the head that you feel you deserve, but bro, you're not an innocent in all of these stories. Shit doesn't just happen *to you to make your life sad and difficult. You might just be responsible for some of it.*

Not this time, asshole. This is not *my* fault. And Kim is a trifling bitch, that much is clear. Fuck your "let's pause and see both sides" bullshit. This is about Katya, my fucking *friend* whom I am capable of being *loyal and trustworthy* to.

Are you really so wrapped up in your own pity-party bullshit that you can't see that, given the way this shitbag world works, Katya wouldn't be at all crazy to believe—

Look. I'm only going to say this once. Then you never speak to me this way again. I've done a lot of shitty things in my life to people I care about. But never have I ever tried to force myself on someone else without their consent. Ever.

That you know of.

Of course, "that I know of."

From your perspective.

Yes.

That's all I'm saying.

Well, you and Kim can ride off into the fucking sunset together, how about that? At the end of the day, her job was pretty easy, huh? Watch from afar all night, don't lift a finger when her friend goes missing, and make a phone call in the morning to make sure that the most monstrous possible demons in Katya's mind all look like me.

Fuck. All I'd wanted to do was help. It was all falling to shit. And I'd been silent on my end of the phone call for far too long.

No matter what was said next, I'd already lost.

"Katya, I don't know what Kim thinks she saw, but that is not true. I bought you one drink, but I would never, *ever* try to take advantage of you like that. You know me. I'd never do something like that to you."

"Yeah, okay," she said quickly. "Listen, I've got to go. I'll talk to you later."

Later came and went.

The grapevine informed me that afternoon that Katya was so angry with me that she never wanted to see me again.

The news made me parched. I poured myself a gin and tonic. Each sip was an urgent relief. I finished my warm-up glass in two minutes, promptly refilled, and collapsed back into my bed, balancing the drink on my comforter. I closed my eyes and a sublime realization found its way to the front of my brain—being a designated driver is the most infuriating, bullshit scam of all time. If my friends had enough money to get wasted at the bar, they had enough money for a cab to get their monkey asses home. And what of these temporary experiments in sobriety? They were nothing more than flimsy attempts to demonstrate self-control to the public—to a bunch of miscreants who, in their own drunkenness, couldn't care less if I could walk a straight line.

I wasn't mending any of the wounds in my broken mind. I hadn't stopped resenting the sun for forcing me into another day. So fuck it.

I'm not so sure that's the appropriate takeaway from this story. Listen, I can feel your anger. I know how you react when you feel aban—

Nope. It's high time you shut the fuck up, because this is my story and I get to decide the morals of my own epic tales. So fuck keeping up appearances. Fuck all of the self-righteous lies I've been telling myself. And motherfuck trying to take care of people who made a *choice* not to take care of themselves.

Fuck all of it.

I downed the remainder of the glass and buried my face in a pillow. The gin had fueled my rage, but the kindling had been there long before, and I wasn't quite sure to whom it was directed. Donning the cape of Sober Party Bro-Mom had left me in puke-stained jeans and robbed of a friend who would never return—significantly more lonely than I'd been twenty-four hours prior.

My eyes shot open in a panic. Sawyer's words from the night before whispered about my mind:

I don't know how to be more lonely than this.

Work made me feel inadequate for thirty hours a day. I was drunk in bed by myself on a Sunday afternoon. Friendships among the damaged, overworked, and scared shitless were proving flimsy. And I was tired—always tired. And alone.

I heard a voice deep in my mind, singing in a ghostly melody: *The pieces of your life aren't loyal. They'll find a way to leave you, they were always borrowed. They'll fly away and watch you fall . . .*

You d— . . . —ve to liste—

Too late. It's all I can hear now. This familiar voice. Haunting me with this melody.

And now it's no longer singing but laughing, lost in a fit of sadistic giggles.

It laughs and it laughs, trailing off into a maddening echo.

So familiar.

Is that me?

What will become of me if I truly do not know how to be more lonely than this?

Track 7: FALLS END

You've been quiet. At least that's how you've been here in your head. Outside, the noise has been nearly unbearable.

I worry when you get this quiet. It's scary in here without you. Especially when I remember what happened the last time you went silent.

I know you hear me. You're writing again, so at least that's something, right? Tell me something. Anything. Make a dumb pun. A crass joke. Let's spar with some witty banter. Or if it's easier, you can just yell at me. I'm pushy. I'm a know-it-all. Call me an asshole for old times' sake. I can take it! Just . . .

Please.

Okay, how about a prompt? That picture that you've been obsessing over. The grainy dark one with words etched into splintering wood: FALLS END.

You wanna tell me where you took it? I can't remember, so that usually means you were pretty drunk. But something about this image cut through the alcohol, huh? Why do y—

Because there are only two ways for falls to end.

Either someone catches you . . . or . . .

Or?

I think it's time for you to go.

No, please. Don't send me back to—

Go.

FOUR

YOU

Dear Z,

I don't know if this is a letter I'll ever send you. But here at the end, as I drown and inhale water with each breath, the only thing I have strength left to do is be honest. Finally. As I spin in this undertow.

Moments come back to me now. Flashes of lightning in a midnight storm. The day we met. You sat two seats down from me, to my left, at a long oak table as we received our new physician orientation. Through each lecture, you snickered at jokes only you could hear.

~~I was hooked. I had to know you.~~ I snickered to myself as I drank you in. Not quietly enough. You threw a playful glance my way.

That was the beginning of us.

The first time we lay sweating, naked next to each other in your bed. I was mesmerized, marveling at each of your slopes and curves while you plucked strands of your hair off my chest. We'd both danced through moments like this before, knew what we shouldn't expect. We worked too closely, slept too little, had not yet mourned the passing of *other loves. Their ghosts nipped at our heels with each step forward. We weren't ready to say the words that would claim each other. We would be friends and distractions.*

Fun. And safe. And harmless.

The simple truths came easily then. I told you that I spoke to my father once every several months and he still never seemed to remember what type of doctor I was. That I had a tendency to sabotage my relationships intricately and persistently so that I always had a built-in exit strategy. That I was nowhere near as kind a person as my smile would have you believe. You told me how ashamed you were of your father for being a spineless coward. That you were equally ashamed of your mother for giving up on happiness decades ago. That saying yes to life's crossroads was infinitely more fun than no. Except for when yes almost got you killed.

Despite our intentions, we'd been building the pillars of intimacy. It was an intimacy that gave me a moment's peace from my nightly blizzard of intrusive thoughts and let a blink of sleep in. An intimacy that straightened my back, lifted my chin high as I trudged through rounds, no matter how often inadequacy stabbed up through my skin from just below the surface.

It was an intimacy that gave me a defiant strength. ~~*A home.*~~ *An oasis in the loneliness. And, after months, it emboldened me to ask if you felt it too. You never knew how scared I always was. Of breaking everything. I've always been so good at breaking things. But what if I didn't? Just this once? The words were a moment from crossing my tongue. You spoke first.*

Your mother had found a lump. A mammogram had agreed. Your mother had just gotten a biopsy.

Your mother had breast cancer.

And although by all accounts it was treatable, your mother had told you to forget about her.

Your mother wanted to die.

Panic. It gripped you tighter with each hollow sound that spilled from your lips: shallow breathing and shortened sentences. Speak for too long, and you'd no longer be able to hold your terror inside. I should have told you then about how well I've known panic.

The real kind. The impending-death kind.

This kind.

It first found me years ago. Fragile teenage hubris shattered on the morning that I learned my own mother had been diagnosed with breast cancer. Panic never spoke. It slid close and I welcomed it. It has a way of embracing; you let it near because it seems so harmless at first, just another nervous pit in your stomach. Then it squeezes, strangles the will from your muscles. Crushes your chest and occludes your windpipe and convinces you that death is the only release.

But I didn't tell you. Didn't tell you how far from alone you were. Because how could I be sure? What did I know of your pain? How could I tell you that your mother hadn't really meant what she'd told you, that she was clawing her way through the stages of grief, mourning the loss of her prediagnosis life? How could I tell you that you were strong enough to become a caretaker to the one who should be taking care of you?

I couldn't. Those weren't truths you'd shared with me yet. They weren't the easy ones.

I could have tried. I wish I had. But the chance that I'd get it wrong seemed too great. If I don't think I can do something right, I usually won't try it at all.

Intricate sabotage, remember?

*So I sat with you in that call room and held your hands
in mine. I told you that I wanted to be there with you
through this, but I wasn't exactly sure how to do it. Perhaps
you just needed someone who would listen. Or maybe you
needed someone to help share the burden of all of the
responsibilities that might fall on you. Whenever you felt
you could, I asked that you tell me how I could support you.
I would do my best.*

You threw my hands away and stood up.
I can't believe that you're trying to make this situation about
you and your needs. How could you be so selfish?

You slammed the door on the way out of the room.

All that rumination and I'd still gotten it wrong.

*I sat there for twenty minutes until my pager went off,
wondering if you were right.*

*You asked me to come over to your house that night.
You'd already had half a bottle of wine. We barely spoke. I
joined you in more wine, which led to sex, which led to
fitful sleep, which led to a lack of focus at work in the
morning, which led to a burned-out brain by shift's end,
which led to more liquor that night. And on it went. For
weeks.*

*You'd mustered the resolve to badger your mother daily
until she finally agreed to the surgery that could save her
life. That stubbornness* ~~that I love about you~~ *paid off. The
night before her operation, as she lay in a hospital bed
complaining to you about the linens, you shot me a text.
Backup needed. Urgently. Before you threatened to kill your
mother quicker than the cancer could.*

*So few things made me smile and laugh in a way that
hadn't been practiced and perfected for show.*

You were always one of those things. ~~You always
will be.~~

It was a slow night on call, so I did come down. You never saw me, but I was there. Seated at a nurses' station, watching you alternate between eye rolls and mischievous smirks as your mother's mouth never stopped moving. The panes of glass and bustle of orderlies and ringing telephones kept me at a safe distance. You'd invited me. Inside. To a moment where you'd no longer hide the truth of the relationship that made you. But I couldn't pass the threshold of that room. It was too intimate. Too close. Too familial. You'd made a mistake, you just didn't know it yet. Every excuse I could think of to deflect the truth: I was a coward. I couldn't calculate how to balance my discomfort, your uncharacteristic moment of vulnerability, and the weight of cancer's deadly shroud.

I couldn't do it perfectly. So I didn't try.

I slipped away.

I hope you're disappointed in me. For justifying all your reasons for being careful.

Maybe you've been disappointed for longer than I think. Maybe you caught a glimpse of my coat rounding the corner out of the unit and chose to save your disgust for later use.

Save it for the next time we drank a night away. It was always easier for you to be ~~yourself~~ vicious ~~and honest~~ on those nights.

I didn't have to wait long.

Drinking to excess in our scant free time was nothing new for the two of us. We found it harmless because the feelings we sought to numb posed no immediate threat. But you started to drink differently in your mother's cancer season. You didn't want to be seen much outside your house anymore. By the time I'd arrive at your door in the evenings, you'd already have beaten me to the bottle by three glasses or more. Our conversations devolved from the mundanities of work to demands that I leave because you could tell that

I didn't want to be there feeling sorry for you. All in an instant.

Who do you think you are? You aren't good enough, Tony. You clearly can't handle being my man, so just go.

I didn't want to accept it then, but you were right: I'm not good enough.

I'd always leave if you asked. You'd call me immediately after. To berate me for not fighting harder to stay.

And by morning, you'd have forgotten the entire thing.

The gaps in your memory left me as the sole witness to your fall.

And I could feel it stripping me into more and more pieces each day.

Your mother survived, but your work wasn't done—the challenges of coordinating the logistics of her recovery and treatments had fallen to you. A responsibility you seemed to resent and savor in equal confusing measure. You squeezed this work in before and after patients. You stopped taking breaks to rest and eat. You'd black out from whatever liquor happened to be in your cupboard each night.

And I enabled you, your descent, with every moment we spent together.

I could feel the night coming where you'd drink yourself into a trip to the emergency room, and I'd have been the one drinking right alongside you.

My breathing was becoming shallower. My sentences shorter.

I knew what that meant. My panic was something I couldn't afford. Neither of us could. Something had to change.

I remember the night I told you that I thought you needed to talk to someone. A professional. We had access to free counseling through the hospital. Here was the phone number. On my own, I wasn't helping you. I couldn't bear

*watching you drown. I'd become your cement boots in the
ocean.*

    In response you looked into my eyes and asked,
So you're saying that you're done with me?

                                                Of course not.
Well, how else am I supposed to see it? You can't handle me
when I'm hurting and just trying to figure things out. And
now you want to pawn me off on a total stranger so that you
don't have to be a part of this anymore, is that it?

    *No, I don't want— Look, I'm just really . . . It feels like
I'm watching you destroy yourself. Every single night. And
I'm helping you do it. And it is terrifying. I just don't want
something . . . irreversible to . . .*

    *The words died on my lips. Couldn't bring myself to
speak the true fears into existence.*

    You turned your gaze to the ground and whispered,
You want to abandon me.

    *You filled your wineglass and hissed at your linoleum
tiles,*
I want you to get out of my house.

    *I left you there. Didn't fight to stay. And I lay awake all
night wishing I had. Intrusive visions of morning sunbeams
falling on your limp body, barely breathing on your kitchen
floor, circled my mind for hours. But I didn't lift a finger to
dial your number. Made the choice not to drive back to you.
To make sure you were safe. Because you'd told me to go.*
~~What kind of man . . . worse, what kind of friend . . . ?~~

    *You sent me a text the next day. I rejoiced. You lived.
Could I come see you after work? I buzzed with anticipation
for the first time in months. That night would be different.
I'd make it different. I had this crazy idea that, for once, I
wasn't resigned to <u>reacting</u> to you. If I wanted things to
change, I could make them change. I'd bring my own*

*provisions: tea or hot chocolate, food made up of actual
nutrients. Maybe suggest a drive with the windows down.
Open air. And we'd see each other with clear eyes for the
first time in weeks.*

You'd love it. I had to believe it was possible.

*I walked through your front door—you always left it
unlocked—and saw an empty wine bottle on your kitchen
table. Candles were lit throughout the living room and down
the hallway. Your voice wafted through the dancing shadows,
humming along to one of your favorite soul records.*

*I found you lying half naked on the floor of the room,
your head leaning against the baseboard, clutching a family
photo album to your chest. You swayed listlessly to Sam
Cooke, eyes blank, an empty wine bottle at your feet. No
awareness of the figure in the doorway, watching the pieces
of what had once been you. Tears fell down your face
without urgency, in a broken, languid stream. And as Sam's
melodies painted a picture of the little tent by the river
where he'd been born, your head sagged, bounced once
before settling on the carpet. Vacant gaze as your lips
mouthed words from somewhere deep in your mind.*

*You know the look: the language of the faces of the dying
when they are tormented by things left undone. We'd both
seen it hundreds of times. But never so far away from the
plaintive monitors and the tubes and the wires and the
machines and the linoleum. Never in the silence of two kids
so starved for love that all they knew was desperation.*

*But there it was: death waiting in the wings of your
glassy eyes.*

No.

You wouldn't be leaving me that night. Not like this.

*So I cleaned up. I pried the empty wine bottle from
between your legs, collected an empty wineglass from the
bathroom sink. Found the pillows, made the bed, and*

grabbed a Merlot-filled coffee cup from the night table. I
placed the glasses in the sink and kicked open your trash bin
to find another empty bottle of red. That made three.

I returned to your side, brushed soggy strands of hair
from your cheeks. You looked at me for the first time.
I can't do this alone anymore.

I know.

I carried you back to your bedroom and laid you on your
stomach with your head just at the edge of the bed, a
wastebasket at the ready just in case your body chose to
reject the evening's liquid nourishment. I lay there next to
you awake all night, listening for each breath. Ready to
jump if any one of them decided to arrive late.

I must have dozed off because I remember waking to
your voice.

What are you doing here?

I looked over at you. Your eyes were clear. And furious.

What do you mean?

I mean how did you get in my bed?

You invited me over last night.

You sat up quickly.

Oh my God, we didn't have sex, did we?

And with that, my mind went to war. With itself. Reason
and betrayal and compassion and rage and misogyny and
hypocrisy and lust and shame and loneliness. Knives out
and sharpened, tearing bloody pieces off one another. I
couldn't be a predator. Never had been. Unless I was?
Maybe not on that night, but hadn't we built sex into a
purely drunken practice? Where did agency live when
neither of us could see straight? Probably in the same place
as consent: nowhere. But I'd just wanted to help. Fuck
that, the only thing I'd helped you do was drink and get
undressed for months. Why should you believe any different
now? Even if we'd been in a relationship? Is that what this

even was? Even if we loved each other? Even then. And who was I kidding? This wasn't love.

Or maybe this was as close as either of us would get.

Who would be believed if we each told our side of our story?

Fuck me, I wouldn't even take my own side.

Snap.

The sound of my brain fracturing. All the questions ceased. All will to . . . anything. It all stopped. All in the space of a moment. Your eyes bored into mine, searching for answers in angry desperation. And where confusion and betrayal and pity and hatred had been etched momentarily into my features, every muscle of expression went slack.

I had nothing left. For you. For me.

I showed myself out.

The ever-present corner of darkness in my mind yawned wide and swallowed me whole as I closed your front door behind me. The sights and sounds of cars, traffic lights, voices, humans—they all passed above, below, and around me. Never close enough to touch, never coming into focus.

I'd been on the road to this place, this void, for months. Maybe years.

I never told you how often I fake feelings. All of the ones that are supposed to be normal. Happiness. Anger. Sympathy. Sadness. I've long since lost touch with how to feel emotions. I don't know why. I suspect it's faulty wiring. My mind doesn't know how to not be broken. I think I hate myself for it. Ha, that might count as the one emotion I've held on to. All of the others? I pretend. And reflect. To keep everyone ~~from asking too many questions~~ ~~getting too close~~ *comfortable.*

And to give myself hope that I might stumble on a kernel of something real by accident. Fake smile enough and I might just remember the spark of something joyful.

That part was never successful. And then it was too late.

Snap. I lost the will to pretend. I felt nothing. Not even hatred for myself.

You came over to my house the next evening because you wanted so badly to know what had happened the night before. You had a sick feeling that it was something bad, possibly irreversible. And my only thought was how interesting it would be for you to feel a new type of pain. What if you could finally see that all of the trauma you'd been drinking away each night was actually spilling out of you, scarring the people you cared about? You might recognize yourself as a monster. And as the only witness on that night, I was in a unique position to help you get there. It was easy. Cold and clinical—a perk of the detachment afforded me by the darkness of the void.

I told you that you'd invited me. I'd walked into your house and found you crying, half naked, on the floor of your guest bedroom. I'd tried to help you to bed, but you pushed me away. Told me to fuck off. I tried again but when I got close, you got more violent: pushing, shoving, slapping, throwing books, hurling wine bottles. Demanding I leave. But I wouldn't go. Not this time. You might hurt yourself by accident, I said. Or worse. I tried to soften the idea of finding a therapist. You could talk to my mom, the psychologist, for free. Fuck that bitch, your mom is a motherfucking cunt, you'd said. And on you went, about my mother and how pathetic she was, what a selfish piece of shit I'd turned out to be, how you didn't need shit from an asshole like me. And with every rage-fueled breath another swing of a bottle, another slap to my face, another unsteady stumble into a kitchen cabinet or near slip on a linoleum floor. At some point you realized that I wasn't leaving despite your best efforts to cut me with words and fingernails and glass. You fell to the ground, heaving violent sobs. I carried you to bed. Cleaned up the mess. Then I joined you. I lay there next to you awake all night, listening for each breath. Ready to jump if any one of them decided to arrive late.

I looked into your eyes at the end of the story and found devastation.

That doesn't sound like me at all.

I said nothing, allowing the false memory to take shape in the lost time of your mind. I regarded you with fascination, as I would a lab rat I'd trapped in an unsolvable maze. You apologized. So many times. You promised that this was it—you needed help, and you were going to find someone to talk to first thing in the morning. I asked if you could leave. I needed some time away from us.

You stopped drinking cold turkey the next day.

I manufactured your rock bottom.

It was emotional abuse, executed to perfection. I took advantage of your vulnerability, lied to you, manipulated you into thinking that you had abused me. But I'd learned from one of the best. You were a master at pulling my strings, convincing me I wasn't worth whatever you had to give.

This was just the long-overdue resolution of a messy, abusive transaction.

Nothing personal. Just business.

Can't call it cruelty without intent.

If I can't care about the outcome, it's just called some shit I did.

I felt no satisfaction that night. No high off a sense of power. No comfort in some great moral victory. No sympathy or empathy for you. No shame or disappointment in myself.

Nothing. Hollow.

Falling.

Falls end.

Somehow.

Another thing I never told you: I hear voices.

In my head.

Probably because I'm crazy.

Not so much distinct voices, as it is an amphitheater-size audience. Sometimes they murmur or laugh, other times they chant and sing. But always, they <u>always</u> celebrate my deficiencies.

Insecurities and pain. They gorge themselves on both.

So it should come as no surprise that they've been particularly fond of you, relentlessly parroting you after you'd call me a regret, or a coward, or the worst thing that ever happened to you. They loved that shit, sang your words gleefully back to me on a continuous loop, day after day, louder every minute.

It's been hell trying to focus through the noise. Impossible to sleep.

Every night with you raised the volume. Made the voices riotous.

Until the night that you forgot.

Snap.

Quiet. The echoes of my self-loathing choir dissipated slowly and gave way to a suffocating stillness. Empty and alone in silence. It smothered me, that silence in the void. It stole my will to fight. For anything.

Suffocation is so much easier if you stop trying to breathe.

And yet even without any fight left in my bones, I held on to a fool's hope of being saved.

There was a day weeks later. I couldn't bring myself to stand up and leave the house. I sent a text asking if you'd come over when you finished work. You wrote back,

*peppering me with questions. Did I need anything? Was
I okay? What could you bring to help me feel better?*

It's amazing how concerned for me you'd learned ~~to act~~
to be over the last several weeks.

*I left all of your questions unanswered. Rolling over in
bed seemed to take minutes, not seconds. I hadn't spoken
a word in over twenty-four hours. Sending you that initial
text message took me forty-five minutes. I'd think about
extending my fingers but find that there was a threshold of
caring about the outcome of the movement that had to be
met before my muscles would even agree to move. An action
potential. Like they taught us in neurology. Any less and I'd
continue to lie still. Locked inside my own body without the
will to search for a key.*

*You arrived that afternoon and found me sitting on the
floor of my bedroom, head lolling against my mattress,
humming the notes to a song I once knew as I stared blankly
out my window. I could feel you standing in the doorway,
watching me.*

*Goddamn. We were mirrors of each other. And neither
one of us had insight enough to notice.*

*You asked me to come downstairs to the living room
when I was ready. I may or may not have nodded my head.
You turned and retreated. I tried for the next twenty
minutes to stand, but I couldn't move a muscle.*

It used to be so easy.

*My front door slammed as you left without another
word.*

*Hadn't I stayed for you? Even when it left me sick and
scarred, hadn't I stayed?*

*I should have known. I wouldn't be saved. Not by you.
You could barely stand to see me like this.*

*I lost hope. I withered unseen. The perfect combination
for casual acts of desperation.*

Cutting yourself is like riding a bike: to start is to be on the edge of falling.

And once you do it, you never forget.

Picking up the knife was easy this time around. None of the momentary apprehension of those first attempts all those years ago. I knew where: the fleshy part of my left hand between my thumb and pointer finger. I knew why: to feel something, anything, that would prove I was still connected to this world. The shock of pain and the trickle of blood jolted me into awareness for a few moments, just enough to get me into my car and on the way to work. As those days went on, my mind would detach, float off into the ether where nothing mattered for minutes on end. The only way to ground myself was to massage my cut until the pain shot through my arm again, and new beads of blood stained my fingers. Such a strange new habit, surely someone would notice? Someone would pull me aside and see the light in my eyes had gone out? Maybe touch my shoulder, or squeeze my hand, or just tell me that swerving through lanes on the freeway with no headlights and no seat belt on the way home from work every night was a bad idea? Because losing me would matter?

Could anybody ~~hear me care for love~~ see me?

No. They couldn't. And you wouldn't. You'd made yourself scarce since the evening that you slunk silently away from me.

I can't blame you. I wouldn't want to watch me fall either.

And so, here I sit. Silence and gin. And a knife. And slow, hollow breaths.

It's amazing how few breaths I need each minute when I don't move. I've been able to get it down to seven.

Sometimes six.

I'm finally writing because this may be goodbye.

> *Finally.*

And I had to type because I can't read my own handwriting anymore.

> *I can't stay on the lines.*
>
> ~~*I love you*~~
>
I don't know if I ever truly loved you. Perhaps I do, and it's that peculiar shade of ~~dependence~~ love between two people who ~~drag each other deeper into the dark~~ hold each other's hands as they both drown.

> *Whatever it is, whatever it was, you deserved the truth before I go.*
>
> ~~*I'm sorry*~~
>
> *And so I go.*

FIVE

FEAR OF FLYING

I came back to the world.

It was all darkness.

A warm breeze lapped the skin of my neck as I breathed deeply and stretched unforgiving muscles. Sand between the toes of my bare feet, soles planted on wooden planks. A dock. I loosened my grip on the railing, dropped my arms to my sides, and leaned forward. Nothing to fear here. I pressed my torso into the wooden beam and craned my neck to greet what lay beyond.

A world bathed in black. No moon to greet me. No stars to guide me home. Only the roar of the ocean beneath, above, and behind me.

The pitch of black. A midnight melody.

Music again, at long last.

The muscles of my face groaned as my lips parted into a smile.

Hazy visions of the last several weeks, disembodied and devoid of context, shot through my mind. Z crying on her bed as I rejected her touch. Some massive failure, the itch of scabbed skin between my fingers, an act of love from afar. The burning relief of alcohol in my chest.

And silence. The crushing silence of every moment in between.

I was in Mexico. On the edge of a dock a quarter of a mile from the shore.

I laughed. The sound died instantly, swallowed by the ocean breeze. My voice was of no use here. What a relief. I laughed even harder. Gratefully. Joyfully. I threw my head back and howled as the wind whistled in my ears.

I was alive.

And I was unemployed.

So. Depression.

It's much more than feeling "the blues," more complex than the sadness that tends to accompany a bad breakup, the emptiness in the wake of losing a job, or even the suffocating array of emotions that typically follows the death of a loved one.

Depression is a medical condition and is defined by a specific constellation of symptoms that can be treated with certain medications and therapies. Given the right (read: awful) circumstances, anyone can plunge into a major depressive episode and struggle to claw their way out for weeks, months, or an entire lifetime.

It's a sneaky bitch of a disease because, like many mental illnesses, it's stigmatized as fuck. Despite its having been studied in depth for ages, there are millions of people who simply don't believe it exists or, if they do, believe it could never happen to them. Because if it did, it would render them vulnerable or weak or crazy in the eyes of everyone they hold dear.

There are quite a few groups of people who tend to feel they can't afford to be perceived like that, mainly because they are already disadvantaged in some way and so have very much to lose. The ones that come to mind quickest for me are Black people. And immigrants.

Also known as my family.

My family has endured and inflicted trauma for so many generations that we've concluded that that's just what family is. Growing up, I'd watch my parents, aunts, uncles, and grandparents spend several hours around the table each Thanksgiving recounting hilarious stories of the creative ways in which their parents had beaten them as kids, of epic public infidelities, run-ins with the police, dehumanizing racist encounters, and domestic violence. They'd all laugh until they cried, then drink something and laugh some more.

We would never ask why things had happened the way they did. And we'd never wonder aloud why we felt it so important to keep telling the same hollow versions of these stories year after year.

Because everyone was fine.

My grandmother who had been in a "bad mood" her entire adult life. My uncle who left his house only once every few months. My other uncle the drug dealer. My grandfather the hoarder and womanizer. Another uncle who, for reasons unknown even to him, refused to travel by airplane. My aunt whose husband had blown his head off with a shotgun.

My father, who spent hours each weekend in front of the television watching horse racing in silence, even as his kids begged for attention.

My mother, who, despite studying human psychology, couldn't

understand why she expected herself to fail at most everything she attempted.

Everyone was *fine*. Doing their best.

Surviving.

It's what they told themselves they had to do in this country. In this world that continually made clear how little it cared about them. In a family that couldn't separate love from pain.

I've only recently learned the vocabulary to identify the various forms of mental illness that run through my family. (It turns out med school was good for something after all.) We've got plenty of abnormal shit going on for sure, but the depression symptom checklist in particular might as well be an admission checklist for our holiday gatherings: abnormal sleep patterns; loss of interest in activities that used to bring joy; feelings of guilt or worthlessness; lack of energy; inability to concentrate; abnormal, unhealthy appetite; psychomotor retardation; suicidal or homicidal ideations. They were all there, in varying combinations and intensities. All there for us to laugh at, no matter how loudly the signs cried out to be recognized. All there to fester and spread and pollute the bloodlines, down both sides of the family and into both my parents.

So where did that leave me?

A textbook taught me that if depression happens to run in your family, a funny thing happens: the further down the family tree you go, the less mentally resilient those individuals tend to be. So when both of your parents (and their parents) have been depressed their entire lives and the tendency toward the disorder swims through your veins, the triggers can be extremely subtle and the onset dangerously insidious—so much so that the characteristics of depression can weave themselves into the tapestry of your personality.

It becomes, simply, who you are.

Who I am.

And then, given enough fuel—enough of the triggers I haven't yet been able to name—depression takes a stranglehold. How do you recognize it? Having grown up surrounded by repressed family members who've built entire lives around their ability to dance around insight into themselves, all while you're held hostage by a disease whose cruelest trick is convincing you it doesn't exist, how do you identify it? Or at the very least notice its unwanted footprints as it seeps into every corner of your mind?

Honestly, it comes down to chance. Motherfucking *luck*.

Maybe a friend or stranger will have the insight to see the pain beneath your bravado and summon the courage to say something. Or maybe you're just not creative, efficient, focused, brave, or weak enough to successfully kill yourself, so you lie awake at night, disappointed by the breaths you continue to take, arrested by a sudden, lucid thought: *These urges are not normal. The fact that they've felt normal for so long is not normal. I can't do this on my own anymore.*

Or neither of those things happens. Fate's coin lands on tails instead of heads, and you end up dead. The story of your life becomes nothing but an agonizing memory in the minds of those who loved you as they flog themselves for never having been able to solve a puzzle they never even knew was there.

Damn.

My eyes widened at these precise, almost academic thoughts as they pushed the roar of the ocean from my mind. For the last several weeks, there had been no witty internal monologue, no self-serving analysis of my day-to-day bullshit. There'd barely even been complete sentences. My mind had been a wasteland of base urges and fuzzy, abstract words and ideas that provided no direction.

Waste. Hunger. Bleed.

Breathe. Flee. Lost.

Live. Leave. Die.

Worth. Less.

I'd become a passenger in my own body, grasping for control in futility, lacking strength and intention. But in the last ten minutes, dormant connections between neurons had sparked apprehensively to life once more—due, most likely, to the slow chemical momentum of something I'd been robotically ingesting for the last fourteen days. Prozac? That definitely sounded familiar. How had I even gotten my hands on that?

I took another deep breath of salty night air, turned, and walked with new deliberation along the dock's creaking wooden planks toward the shore. With each step, more fragmented memories came cascading from all corners of my mind, snapping into sequence.

I had a sinking feeling that this was going to be a movie I didn't want to watch.

I never sent the letter to Z. Probably because I could no longer see the value in sharing it. I was a lost cause with a nasty cutting habit, rotting on my apartment floor every evening, contemplating suicide in my catatonia. She didn't need the details or the half-hearted apologies or the obscured cries for help. Nobody did.

She'd gone radio silent for a few days—very unlike her, as we'd texted daily for months, even in our worst moments—then chimed in with a cheerful Friday afternoon invitation: in recognition of and response to my "rough patch," she thought the two of us could run away for a weekend, escape the hospital's stranglehold, get massages, boil in a hot tub, whatever I wanted. Exclamation points. Smiley emojis.

I texted back several hours later. Promptness and consideration were no longer in my toolbox.

"No. Had to leave. Got in the car this afternoon and headed south. Not sure where I'll end up."

She bombarded me immediately with four straight phone calls that I sent directly to voice mail. Panicked text responses pinged from my phone: *Where are you? Please pick up. Tony, please answer me. Are you safe? Did you hurt yourself? Where are you? Please pull over and call me. I won't be able to sleep tonight if I don't hear from you. Please?*

"I'm safe," I finally responded. "Need to get away from everyone. You can sleep."

Of course, I hadn't meant to get away from *everyone*. I'd accepted another girl's offer of companionship that weekend and had driven to meet her in West Virginia. We'd met at a house party months back while she was visiting Michigan for a weekend, and had nothing in common but loneliness and a desire for meaningless sex, which was just as well, seeing as I had nothing else left to give. I left Z to panic alone as I drank liquor with strangers in a Charleston bar. Typed the words "I'm safe" into the face of my phone as I slipped away into the frosty Appalachian night.

"Need to get away from everyone."

My feet led me away from the bustling main street, down alleyways, across train tracks, into the stillness of a forest. I followed the sound of rumbling fresh water. The dewdrops on tips of wild grass slowly dampened the thin canvas of my Chuck Taylors.

Entranced by the echo of water that reverberated through the shaved foothills of coal country, I missed all of the subtle signs that I was approaching the edge. I stopped abruptly as the moon emerged from low-lying clouds, and the echoes deepened before me. A gorge yawned wide just beyond my feet. A comforting warmth surged through me. How peaceful it could be to admit defeat and leave the swirling, intrusive, self-loathing whispers in my wake as I swan-dived into the darkness beyond the bedrock.

"You can sleep."

A gust of wind set me off balance.

I could have let it take me.

Instead I dropped to the ground, limbs spread-eagle, flat against the last few feet of solid ground before the fall.

You can still go.

My mind had been silent for weeks, save this one voice. It was never welcome. But I never sent it away.

Not today, I replied.

It would be so easy. You don't even have to jump. Just let the wind take you.

I can't, I shot back. I scratched into the frozen earth with every fingernail, desperately searching for purchase as brittle leaves whipped past my face.

What are you holding on to? They'd all be better off without you. Be selfless for once in your life. Be brave.

I squeezed my eyes shut and shook my head against the twigs, not to rid myself of the voice but to ward off the truth it knew. The truth that gave it strength and leached my resolve.

Oh, that's right, you've never been brave. It howled with laughter, amplified by the wind. *Coward. You'd rather just be careless with your life. Careless until something destroys you by accident.*

Because the bad things, the failures, they're never your fault, are they? Never anything you'd take responsibility for. You never make them happen. They all just <u>happen to you</u>.

Please leave, I pleaded. *Why can't I make you go away?*

Because your heart isn't in it. You want me here. You need the reminders of who you really are. So no matter how sick I am of your fucking existence, I'm trapped here with you. For a supposedly smart guy, you are so dumb. And so stubborn. And so useless. I just have to laugh.

I opened my eyes, let a breath burn my chest, and surrendered. The voice was right. It always was.

Since you're clearly not going to do anything exciting, why don't you get up and get out of here? Maybe you'll get your wish and get crushed by a drunk driver tonight. You won't even have to think about it. Over in an instant. Unless you suffer. Now <u>that</u> would be hilarious.

The solitary snickering echoed as I got up and marched back through the West Virginia grass. I looked down once more at my phone and hit send.

For nine hours, my phone remained idle, no messages in or out. Then, as the familiar industrial skeletons of the Midwest rolled past my windows on my drive back to Michigan, a single message pinged. It was from Z: "Hey, did I leave my pants at your place last night?"

I read the sentence three times, just to be sure I wasn't hallucinating. I hadn't been the only one searching for a pressure-release valve that weekend, it would seem. Unexpected but not surprising. I drove on without anger. Not even a shred of curiosity.

She checks on you just to ease her own conscience. But she knows what I know: you're not worth the fight.

I haven't been worth much to anyone.

Will you let her leave? Will you fight?

What's the point? She's already gone. They always go.

Just as you expect them to.

Just as I always expect them to.

My seat belt started to feel a bit tight. I took it off for the rest of the drive home.

That evening we sat in Z's bedroom in the fading light of dusk. She'd coiled herself against the headboard, knees pulled tightly in to her chest. I perched on the bed's edge, eyes downcast, exhausted by the effort it took to breathe in enough air to support a voice any louder than a whisper.

"We need to let each other go."

I said it. Croaked it. My voice had reached an unsettling state of disrepair.

"Tony, no," Z said through the wild nest of hair that had fallen over her face. "Please just let me in. Even a little bit. You didn't leave me when I was lost." The bed shifted and her arms found their way around my chest from behind and held on with a tender resolve I'd never felt from her before. "I don't want to leave you. Not like this."

She's already gone. Smart girl!

"I didn't leave you," I said. "And look where that's fucking gotten us."

I unfolded her arms and stood. She cried. Her arms, suddenly in search of something to hold, pulled her knees in again.

She gathered herself, keeping her gaze on the floor. She had a funny habit of avoiding my eyes when the truth was looming. "But I love you."

She doesn't!

She looked so small in the fading light. Her body didn't quake as she wept. She swayed dreamily, as if she were in a trance, her knees glistening with her steady tears.

"I love you too."

I walked out of the room and heard her erupt into wails of grief as I opened her front door and stepped over the threshold for the last time.

She'd be fine. She'd already found herself another shoulder to cry on.

I picked the scab on my left hand that night and gouged a fresh wound with my favorite kitchen knife. I was suddenly very tired. I let the blood drip down to my fingertips as I made my way to bed. Each day the blood ran from my hand for a little longer. I must have been cutting deeper. Flirting with the arteries I knew to be millimeters from the knife's edge.

One careless cut and I'd finally rest.

I watched with heavy eyelids as a dark stain spread into my pillowcase for several minutes. The spread stopped. Clots dutifully formed in the deep layers of my raw, lacerated skin.

Too bad, I thought, no accidental release today.

I closed my eyes and slept a coward's sleep.

Wooden planks gave way to cool grains of sand as I reached the shore. In the darkness my feet groped for the damp traces of low tide on the beach. I sat to face the ocean once more. And I listened. Hard. Probed my mind for any hint of a whisper. Any echoes of an unwanted voice between my ears.

Nothing. No one. Silence and the ocean breeze.

I wanted to rejoice in relief, but I couldn't trust the quiet. I'd never experienced peace this profound, this absolute. It had to be just a matter of time before the fallen angel on my shoulder spit poison into my ear.

But until then, my mind was my own. For once. Maybe for the first time. It was beautiful. Like waking up.

I closed my eyes and let the cool, salty mist wash over my face. My brow furrowed as I felt the flood of more lost moments pouring in. I readied myself for another reckoning, and the rising tally of how much I'd lost.

My memories of the preceding few weeks (months?) at work as a junior ENT resident were unnervingly indistinct. The days had passed as if they'd been soaked in tears—an undulating world of abstract shapes and colors. Faces animated before my eyes with streaked features and dulled edges, blobs of sepia tones in motion. With my perception impaired by a malfunctioning brain, there was much that I simply could not see, including just how bad I was at my job. And I was only getting worse.

Each morning my muscles required more and more convincing to creak into action. As a result, I was late to morning rounds every day, and eventually I no longer saw the point of making excuses. Judging by the way the chatter of patient presentations didn't skip a beat when I'd finally trudge through the resident room door, my excuses held no weight for my coworkers either. They'd stopped expecting better of me.

My patient assessments and plans became lighter and more concise by way of my worsening tendency to omit crucial details. Any pride I might have felt in finally cracking the "get more effi-cient" code was trashed when I realized I'd traded "Tony's too slow at his job" for "Tony fucked up today's surgical schedule because he didn't tell us that the patient has an uncontrolled bleeding disorder." Concentration was a job requirement. And with my world quickly becoming nothing but blurred edges, the minutiae were lost. I literally could not see the details.

Perhaps the most alarming change (to me, at least—my colleagues didn't give a shit) was my sudden inability to put on a show. No matter the emotional turmoil or uncertainty, I had always been able to hide behind a high-wattage smile and a booming laugh. If you were to ask my high school buddies or, hell, even my fucking parents what I was like as a teenager, they'd remember Tony as happy-go-lucky. A constant source of Disney Channel–level sunshine even as my parents stumbled through a messy divorce and my mother vomited through chemotherapy. I convinced myself that the image of a perfectly happy, perfectly smart, perfectly *complete* kid was what the world wanted from me. It was a persona that had the power to ease others' burdens. To save relationships. To keep families together. And it came so easily. I became so facile at putting on the mask that I'd often forget I was wearing it. On a good day, in the mirror I could even fool myself.

But here in this Detroit linoleum fortress, bruised and battered by what Z and I had called "love," sleep deprived, regularly waking to urine-soaked sheets, perpetually hungover and bleeding more often than not as illness and death waited impatiently beneath every pager siren, my mask had finally cracked and fallen to pieces. It had become too difficult to maintain. And without it I was a dried-out husk, fully exposed, with no cartoonish joy to offer.

Not only had I lost the fake smiles, but my connection to the world around me—my ability to relate to anyone outside my own head—was gone in what felt like an instant. Other people's faces no longer made sense to me. When I sat across from patients, I couldn't decipher what wide eyes or furrowed brows or sneering lips were trying to tell me, so my responses lacked any shred of empathy or emotional intelligence. That's actually a core trait of psychopaths, so I was in really healthy company.

And the voices in my head were getting much more confusing. My increasingly bold and sadistic antagonist was having a grand old time, never missing an opportunity to parrot my bosses' and senior residents' dismissive asides and casual insults back to me multiple times a day. But sometimes beneath his commanding voice I'd catch barely audible fragments of derisive whispers. I couldn't understand what they were saying exactly or tell from which direction they'd originated, but I could *feel* their shit-talking energy. And they seemed to be loudest behind closed doors at work. With each answer I didn't know and each detail I omitted, the air around me became increasingly charged with secrecy. I felt the weight of hastily finished whispers as I walked into rooms to greet my coworkers, nearly choked on the polluted silence that followed as I did my work, and tried my best to block out the snickers that filled the air as I left and shut the door.

Instead of reaching out and helping me get back on track, residents and attendings alike had opted to share hushed jokes behind my back.

Or maybe it was all in my head? I had a history of hearing things, after all.

I mean, the whispers I thought I had been hearing walked in lockstep with the sentiments of my chronic inner soliloquy. They were almost *too* conveniently aligned.

Maybe I was just going fucking crazy.

Or maybe no one asked if I was okay because, in their minds, I'd finally achieved a long-awaited milestone: to the naked, medically trained eye, I was finally adopting a more serious demeanor. I wasn't getting attached to my sob-story patients. I was keeping an appropriate emotional distance from the work: prescribing and treating and cutting and sewing with cold indifference.

In short, I was finally starting to act like a surgeon.

M y eyes went wide, my heart quickened, and my fingers grasped for purchase in the brittle grains of sand. I was in Mexico. I was not in Detroit. It was Wednesday. Why the hell wasn't I at work?

"Fuck," I whispered to the rolling black clouds. "I failed it."

T wo days after I walked out of Z's house, I sat for an eight-hour exam.

It was Step 3: the final feature in the medical trainee licensing trilogy that had plagued me since my anxious days in Atlanta. I'd meant to study. For months it had been on my to-do list, but there always seemed to be a reason to put it off: long day at work, too tired; Hae Won wanted a partner to share his weed as he watched basketball; Z needed me, always needed me; other residents joked over lunch about how easy the test had been when they'd taken it a month ago.

Push it, put it off, procrastinate. Then panic. Then do the thing. Then do miraculously well and learn no lessons. Or do poorly and find anything and anyone but myself to blame.

I'd done this dance hundreds of times in my life. It had become a reliable harbinger of my major depression episodes. Let enough responsibilities slip and I'd convince myself that I had no control of my life, and then I'd give up.

Damn. Insight. Where the hell has this been all my life?

I didn't study at all for the test. I showed up and, for hours, clicked answers at random, shifted uncomfortably in my chair, picked at my fresh scabs and itched to crawl into a dark space far away from the shifty eyes of self-assured test takers and fluorescent lights.

I failed the shit out of that test. And this time, I didn't place any blame. Why put the onus on anyone or anything when the test meant nothing to me? What did another failure matter?

As it turns out, it mattered a lot.

The General chortled in mirthless disbelief when I called to inform him of my test results. In all his years he'd never known a resident to fail Step 3. I was setting new records in underachievement. Awesome.

I'd been on the cusp of beginning my third year of training, but I'd go no further, he told me. Until I had retaken the test and passed, I would be taking a leave of absence.

No more paychecks. No more day job.

I begged various family members until I managed to cobble together the nine hundred dollars to reregister for the test, studied listlessly for a week, and retook it without a shred of confidence. That was last Friday. I wouldn't receive the results for a month.

A month alone. No patients. No money. No Z. No will for self-preservation.

If ever there was a recipe for my death, that was it.

As if she could feel my desperation from hundreds of miles away, my mother dropped a thousand dollars into my bank account that night. No conditions, no strings, only a brief note attached: *Take this. Find a beach somewhere. Quiet your mind.*

I hadn't ever told her the truth of how I'd been disintegrating. It would only serve to scare her. But she'd read between the lines of my robotic, truncated texts and emails. She sensed something was amiss in how often I'd miss calls and how rarely I'd return them.

Sometimes moms just knew.

And this time it might just have saved my life.

Fuck.

Just a few days ago I wanted to end my life.

And it wasn't the first time I've wanted to.

Just the first time I dared admit it.

I took a job right out of college as a high school teacher at a private school in rural Massachusetts. I had no teaching degree, but they figured a Harvard kid was smart enough to figure it out. They paid me to teach and live on the campus as a dorm parent to the boarding students. It was the loneliest year of my life to that point. Not because teaching was hard—I knew how to do it, and the kids and their parents loved me—but because half of the faculty would take time out of their days to try to convince me that I was bad at it. Every day. For a year.

My friends were an hour's drive away. My family was about three. My girlfriend and I were on the rocks, slowly and painfully creating very different lives for ourselves in the way that college sweethearts tend to do. And one morning, on my way back to my dorm apartment after a particularly strained weekend with the lady friend, I pushed the speedometer to eighty miles per hour on the Mass Pike and just . . . let go of the wheel.

I drifted left. Across one lane. Two. Horns blared. I came back to myself as my tires thudded over uneven pavement and I swerved to avoid the stone divider separating me from oncoming traffic. I pulled over in the hazard lane to catch my breath, but it continued to race in and out of my chest. I dialed 911 with clammy, clumsy fingers and ended up in the emergency room.

Panic attack, they said. Go see a psychiatrist.

I didn't fight it. That morning on the highway had felt at once terrifying, exhilarating, and somehow inevitable. I knew none of that could be normal. So I sat across from the doctor, expecting to navigate a deep psychological dive, only to give curt answers as he rattled off a checklist. *Was I having trouble sleeping?* I've never slept well, so these days were no different. *Trouble concentrating at work?* No, I could get my lesson plans done fine. *Had I thought about killing myself? Did I have a plan?* Never. I'd just been careless.

Depression and anxiety were his diagnoses, though I honestly felt like I'd aced the questionnaire. I went home with two bottles of pills. The antidepressants would take a couple of weeks to kick in, so in the meantime I'd been instructed to take a few of the anxiety pills each day. Benzodiazepines. Such funny drugs. They blunt the body's physical response to stress. So even though my brain continued to dive into sudden bouts of panic, my heart and lungs maintained a steady rhythm, my fingers didn't shake, and my thoughts got cloudy and disorganized. My body refused to freak out even though my mind was begging it to. The more I pleaded, the slower my body seemed to move. The deeper my desperation, the less I felt.

That's the first time I picked up a knife. Not to kill myself. Just to hurt myself. A little bit. Just to make sure I could still feel something. Anything.

No intent to kill. No plan. Just a speeding car adrift on a

highway and bloody cutlery in the sink. Those thoughts didn't count as suicidal. They couldn't.

I was so sure.

The second time I wanted to end my life was . . . Well, I actually already shared it in these pages a couple of years ago. Incompletely. So much for honesty. I was just so heavily fucking ashamed of myself that . . . Goddamn. That self-loathing apprehension feels so inconsequential now.

My last year of medical school in Atlanta wasn't all manic drinking and rampant misogyny and the creation of enough noise to drown out the derisive chorus in my head. The loss of Sarah from my life—actually, the *rejection* of Sarah from my life—had left me devastated. Even though I was the one who'd ended it, I couldn't shake the feeling that I was a failure for not being able to make it work, which . . . might be a pattern for me in relationships? There were definitely shades of those same feelings present throughout the life I'd built around Z. The point is that the loss of Sarah ate away at me far more than I ever dared admit.

Add to that the loss of control and constant dread that I'd fucked up my future before it had even gotten started that the looming Match provided, and I had created the perfect playground for my head voices to paralyze me. And of course, given the opportunity, they did. In the weeks before Match Day, I started showing up late to my pediatric surgery rotation in the hospital. The rationalizations flowed freely: this was widely known as one of the easiest rotations of med school—it barely required any work to pass; my grade didn't matter, as my Match application had already been turned in; they didn't need me at the hospital, my useless ass couldn't even place orders in the computer; there were plenty of other students passing through, they probably wouldn't even notice if I wasn't there on time.

Lateness turned into absence. My absences weren't spent partying or chasing girls.

I was in my bed. Unable to pull myself out for hours. Unwilling to answer the telephone. Sipping from the bottle I kept on my nightstand. Counting how few breaths I could manage each minute.

And, of course, retrieving my old friend from the silverware drawer.

The feelings were similar enough to what I'd navigated during my teaching stint that I managed to pull myself out of bed long enough to get to an appointment with University Student Health. I told the nurse practitioner that I'd been cutting myself, that I didn't care if I was alive or dead but, since I didn't have a formal plan for how or when I was going to kill myself, I was told it didn't count as *seriously* suicidal. The NP felt fine with sending me home with a new prescription for antidepressants. She offered me benzos for anxiety too, but I was too scared of what they might do to me this time around.

So I went back to my bed and stayed there for days, trying to ignore the new hourly urges to put my death on the day's schedule. I wondered if the NP would have taken this new development seriously. I guess I should have called for another appointment, but my drive for self-preservation had been exhausted. She'd missed her chance to help me.

After a couple of weeks, my head began to clear. Medicine works, I guess. I woke up one Monday morning. On time. I got dressed and was about to head in to the hospital when I realized that my pediatric surgery rotation had ended a week ago.

I'd failed it. Insufficient attendance.

The consequence? I wouldn't graduate on time. I'd receive my diploma only after I'd made up the rotation, and I couldn't do that until after our official graduation day.

The administration took pity on me and, in an effort to quell my humiliation, let me dress and walk the graduation stage with my classmates. I received the same big blue diploma folder as everyone else on that day. Except mine was empty. I kept the secret from most of my family. All of my friends. I posed for fraudulent pictures and accepted undeserved congratulations. And wished I'd been far more daring and careless with my kitchen knife.

The tide crept higher in the light of the late-night moon, burying my toes deeper in the sand with each retreating wave. Somehow the minutes passed and my mind remained my own. No intruders. Just me. And a curiosity I'd never entertained before.

Now that I'd played back each of these dark seasons, I wondered if maybe there'd been some unifying themes. Recurring triggers that reliably torpedoed my ability to cope. Convinced me that my body deserved to be punished. Stole my belief that life was worth living.

I closed my eyes. Sank into the music of the night as I let the words find me.

Inadequacy.

Inadequacy and abandonment.

There'd always been some failure to reach a goal I knew I should have been able to achieve. And my first instinct after coming up short was always to take it as an indictment of my worth.

There had always been someone close to me. Someone I cared deeply for. Maybe even loved. And I always left them. Abandoned them before they could abandon me, even if they never showed any sign that they would.

And then I'd always unravel.

Always get lost.

Shit.

I think it's time that I properly introduced my father.

I've never known much about the likes and dislikes of Anthony Lloyd Chin-Quee. The ones that mattered, anyway. One detail I do know: he could not abide the cold. So on the February day of his arrival from Jamaica in 1970s New York City, when he gazed, bewildered, at a landscape completely at odds with the images of America he'd seen on *Leave It to Beaver*, his disillusionment took on painful physical form as the freezing wind took root in his bones. He found no whimsy in the sight of his breath hanging in the air. No charm in the charcoal-colored dregs of week-old snow. Winter in the States was stubborn. Stagnant. Oppressive. And at odds with everything he'd ever known the warmth of the sun to allow.

Just two nights prior, he lay awake on a dormitory cot. The order for "lights out" initiated, as usual, energetically whispered teenage discourse: adolescent politics, jokes at the emotional expense of friends and enemies, and all of the other things boys talk about as they navigate the anxiety of becoming men. But Anthony Lloyd Chin-Quee lay silent that night. Embraced by the warm tropical breeze, entranced by the light of the moon as it peeked through distant clouds, he was content.

He'd never known much about stability. He never knew his father: the man had disappeared from his life before he had learned to walk. But he didn't desert his family without leaving a keepsake. Anthony Lloyd Chin-Quee and his siblings were victims of their father's genes and had all inherited physical features that made "others" of them. In a sea of sun-kissed brown faces, he stuck out like a sore East Asian thumb. Try as he might to fit in, his friends on that little Caribbean island were always sure to classify him as *Chynee-man*.

A *whuh mek yuh skin suh yellow?*

Anthony Lloyd Chin-Quee never had an answer. The man who had made him *so yellow* had abandoned him before he could ask questions.

His mother left a few years later, on a plane to America in search of a better life. Once she'd saved enough money, she'd send for as many of her four children as she could afford and they'd join her in the States. In the meantime, she left them all in the care of a neighbor. For years. The children would receive a letter from their mother at the High Holidays. Easter and Christmas. Season's greetings. Working as a housekeeper in a hotel. Make sure you go to church and do your schoolwork.

So Anthony Lloyd Chin-Quee grew taller. His voice deepened. And as the years went by, he'd think of his mother only in passing. He knew that he appreciated her sacrifices for her children. He just didn't know her personally.

Boarding school was a relief.

Living in a community of boys his age on equally orphaned footing for months at a time. Under a secure roof. Meals on time. And a bed by the window through which the moon kissed him good night. For once, his life wasn't shifting constantly beneath his feet.

A gentle hand shook him awake. His dorm parent stood over him, speaking in hushed tones as the rest of the room slept.

Wake up and pack everything. You leave tonight.

Your mother is here. She's taking you straight to the airport.

In that instant Anthony Lloyd Chin-Quee's life in Jamaica evaporated. He arrived in Bushwick, Brooklyn, a few hours later. Uprooted and unmoored once more, he was in painfully familiar territory. Except this time he was an immigrant. And it was fucking freezing.

The tiny fingers of Anthony Lloyd Chin-Quee's firstborn son grabbed at his beard for the first time on a crisp autumn morning in 1983.

The weight of his American life bore down on him in waves in those first joyful, terrifying moments. He'd managed to carve out a piece of the American dream for himself in the ten years since he'd arrived. A high school diploma and a college degree. He passed the New York State bar exam because that's what you did if you were a West Indian immigrant and didn't have the grades to be a doctor: you became a lawyer. Met a girl, got dumped by a girl, got kicked out of the house by his mother for being too much of a bummer. Met another girl while on the rebound. This one was kind and quiet and had learned to hide her intelligence, opinions, and ambitions. Mixed messages from her own "proud" West Indian parents. He married this girl because . . . well, it was time. At the geriatric age of twenty-seven, he was over the hill. Time to settle down. And so a year later, Anthony Lloyd Chin-Quee first laid eyes on me. Introduced me to the world as his namesake. He had so much to teach me. And I was an unwritten open book.

Anthony Lloyd Chin-Quee went to work every day at a modest law office that bore his own shingle. He never dealt in checks or credit cards. All business was conducted in cash. It was simpler that way, he told his wife. More secure. But curiously, most of that cash never made it home to his family. It was a puzzle my young mind couldn't solve. Daddy was a lawyer. Lawyers make money. So why did Mommy line up at a government office one day, only to turn around and walk home, eyes to the pavement, having realized she was too ashamed to apply for food stamps even though food in the cabinets was quickly running out? Why were tales of break-ins at Daddy's office as reliably commonplace as the changing of the seasons? And why did I answer the door one night to find a man looking for my father, barely concealing an aluminum bat behind his back, and know instinctively that I had to lie about his whereabouts? I didn't know. So I asked. My father never answered. But he did once take me on a field trip to the horse-racing track. We sat on bleachers as the trained beasts thundered past, and we spoke of shoes. Every kid needed a new pair of sneakers at the beginning of the school year. But what was the only thing better than one pair of shoes? Ten pairs! And so, he explained, he was laser focused every day on turning one pair of shoes into ten. As quickly as possible. For his family. Sure, sometimes he'd end up with no pairs, or owing a pair to someone else. And that was okay—walking around in your socks is fine for a little while. But he knew with certainty that ten pairs were coming soon. Right around the corner. Maybe even fifty. Or one hundred pairs! Someday soon, we wouldn't want for shoes ever again. He promised.

And so Anthony Lloyd Chin-Quee taught me responsibility.

One development he did not anticipate at the outset of his journey into fatherhood was his wife's discovery of her own voice. She'd spent a lifetime strangled into silence by her parents, but the existence of her children demanded more of her. So she demanded more of him. She was the first person in his life to call him an addict. The truth of it threatened his ego and sent him retreating into a corner of his fragile mind, raging all the way. The arguments grew steadily louder each night until their voices shook the walls and rattled the springs of their son's bed, jolting him awake. My mother pleaded. He needed help. She'd help him find it and support him through it. But Anthony Lloyd Chin-Quee didn't have a problem. She switched tactics: *What's the plan for paying the overdue mortgage?* He'd get it, he replied. *But how? Tell me exactly how.* Once again he found himself trapped. Cornered. So he lashed out. Self-preservation over all else. His footsteps pounded. He roared, "You know, sometimes I think you've dropped straight down to hell!" Their bedroom door exploded open, spilling light onto his son's face.

Twenty feet away, the boy sat bolt upright in his bed, his chest heaving. In the eyes of his son, Anthony Lloyd Chin-Quee caught a glimpse of what he had become: a beast, a clawing, frothing, bloodthirsty nightmare. He approached his son's doorway carefully, saw the boy tense beneath his sheets. Maybe he'd be able to explain how he was a victim. How his wife's words, not his actions, were the work of the devil. How there was nothing to fear and that everything would be all right.

But no words came. He'd done enough lying for one night.

He reached for the knob, whispered *I love you* into the darkness as shadows washed over his son's face, and closed the door.

His marriage was not long for this world. But before the divorce paperwork was done and dusted, Anthony Lloyd Chin-Quee had already found someone new. To be alone, partnered only with his increasingly dark thoughts—no, he wouldn't go into that. He had to believe that he'd just fallen hopelessly in love and had no choice in the matter. So he sat me down and told me that he'd prematurely started dating. She was great. I'd love her when I met her.

But for now, I should keep it to myself. Because I was the man of the house now that he'd be gone. And men kept secrets.

He got remarried a couple of years later to the same secret woman. She was several years his junior. He shrugged off her immaturity, jealousy, and speech impediment and instead basked in her simplicity. She just wasn't that smart. She rarely asked questions, and when she did, he could dance around them with dicey logic and confident delivery. She was just *easier* than my mother. What a relief.

I was a teenage groomsman at the wedding, sweating bullets in my rented tuxedo in the humid summer heat. He locked eyes with me for a moment when he arrived at the altar. Inscrutable as always. I lowered my eyes as anger and disgust pulsed in my ears and listened to him promise to have, hold, and cherish just one person until his death. For the second time in his life.

And so Anthony Lloyd Chin-Quee taught me that love was a transaction. Bought and sold. Given and taken away. Never forever.

We spoke only sporadically over the ensuing years. Birthdays, High Holidays, college graduation, requests for spending money in lieu of the child support that he never sent. His shame kept him silent, and my anger kept me pretty fucking angry. Then one weekend as I cruised through Atlanta on a blooming spring afternoon free from medical school responsibilities, my phone buzzed in the cup holder. I answered Anthony Lloyd Chin-Quee's call. He got straight to the point. He'd recently begun attending meetings where the participants remained anonymous. The time had come to admit the truth to himself. And once he did, he was compelled to apologize to those he'd hurt on his journey to the bottom. It was a small step. One of twelve, in fact. But he was committed to making amends.

I didn't believe him. But I tried. Because I always wished I could believe him.

He called a few more times over the next few weeks, searching blindly for footholds into my life. He was persistent, I'd give him that. I'd even allow that his effort was admirable. But no sooner had that consideration crossed my mind than my phone rang. News from my mother. An argument had erupted between my father and one of my two younger brothers. My brother had requested that my father not bring his new wife to his college graduation. She had never been supportive of him, he explained, and her presence would be painful. All of Anthony Lloyd Chin-Quee's recent practices of understanding imploded in an instant. He didn't think. He reacted. In a rage. Which sparked a matching rage within my brother. The two men had always been too similar. In the end, my father refused to attend his son's college graduation at all. My youngest brother attempted to visit my father in person to broker peace and plead for understanding. But he and my father had always been too different. There was no compassionate common ground to be found. My father barricaded himself in his house. His wife barked my brother off their front porch.

My family—the ones who'd stayed, the ones who'd been abandoned—was under attack. My instincts of self-preservation went out the window. Regardless of what it meant for my well-being, it was time to stand. I picked up the phone. Anthony Lloyd Chin-Quee answered.

His fury at my brother screamed through the tinny speaker, but I would have none of it. He wasn't angry with me, and I told him if we were to have a conversation, he'd keep his voice under control. He felt trapped once again, backed into a corner by his shame. Because he knew, despite the words he stammered, that my brother wasn't being childish or petty. Amends did not erase the pain he had caused. He knew that he was living the consequences of his lifetime of mistakes. And it did not feel very good at all.

I told him all of this. He sputtered and stuttered, scratching for a way to refute me. But the truth had stripped him naked.

So he hung up on me.

When the line went dead, I broke down, shuddering desperate sobs into my palms, completely spent by the emotional effort it took to parent my father. And I was consumed by my own foolishness for believing in him, even for a moment.

And so Anthony Lloyd Chin-Quee taught me that people don't change.

Months later, he sat across from me for the first time in years. Uneasy small talk gave way to charged silence, each of us convinced he was the shattered mirror image of the other. My father had found himself on the receiving end of a letter from me a few weeks earlier. It was devastating in its formality—an efficient dressing-down of his life choices, dripping with poised anger and disappointment. I had started seeing a therapist, and I had reasoned that the first step toward the exorcism of my pain was to share it. If I didn't start now, my mind would rust and erode, just like a certain gambling addict I knew. Anthony Lloyd Chin-Quee read the letter in silence as the familiar, protective rage bubbled. But with nobody around to victimize, he turned the anger on himself. His son had eclipsed him in every way but still found himself trapped by a desire to hope for and believe in a father who didn't believe in himself. There had to be something he could do or say to set me free.

So he got on a plane to Atlanta and arrived on my doorstep. And when the time came to break the silence, he searched inside himself for bravery and found nothing. He groped for words of reassurance that he could and would do better, but they never came. Tears fell from his eyes in a steady stream as he looked into my own, and he decided that the merciful thing to do would be to extinguish the glimmer of hope that I had held on to so desperately all of these years. No more promises or platitudes. No more lies. All that remained was a simple truth that he hoped would liberate us both.

"I'm sorry that I failed you as a father."

And so Anthony Lloyd Chin-Quee taught me to give up.

The tide was coming in. I knelt on all fours in the wet sand, watching my hands bury themselves deeper with the wash of each extinguished wave, consumed by the ridiculous realization that I'd just recited my father's unauthorized biography to an audience of one.

And I didn't even know if half of it was true.

I'd pieced it together from facts I'd stolen: anecdotes around tense family dinner tables, whispered conversation fragments, loaded glances and sobbing confessions. But rarely from the man himself. And his motivations? His reasons? All blanks that I'd filled in on my own.

And the fact that that's all I'd been given? That I'd grown up with an absentee father who slept just a few feet away and understanding him had fallen to me because he refused to try to understand himself?

It made something shift inside me. I tipped out of balance.

My head felt a bit too light, my breaths too shallow. Panic's familiar signature. But only for a moment. My body was grounded in the shifting sands. My senses sharpened by the salty air and churning sea. My skin, my muscles, my eyes burned with an unfamiliar heat. This was no panic attack. This was anger. This was fury. And it felt fucking incredible.

I'd spent a lifetime tamping it down, convincing myself that my anger wasn't healthy. That it was, in fact, useless. I had to believe that. Because if I didn't, if I admitted that I'd been simmering with rage every day of my life because of him and I finally let it erupt, I might never wrangle it back in. And if I couldn't control what I became after that, I'd succumb to the thing I feared most.

That's why I built the mask. It's why I taught myself to smile and listen and laugh. It's why I achieved. Why I showed the world that I could be excellent. If perfection existed, I could embody it.

I'd be more than he could ever be.

I needed to keep it up. I needed to believe that with enough effort and enough time, I could make it more than just a facade. Because I knew that, just beneath my skin, my father lived inside me. He lived in my insecurities and my weaknesses. He lived in my fears.

I hated myself for it.

And if I let the full measure of that hatred and all of the years of anger erupt? I'd finally face the truth: I was just like him.

It was genetics. It was in my blood.

It was inevitable.

Fuck it. So be it. I had nothing more to lose.

I'd never let myself scream so loud. As the world slept and the wind carried my cries out to sea, I bellowed my vocal cords raw. I howled on, guttural and primal, as my muscles shook in defeat and jagged breaths threatened to overtake me.

I screamed until I realized I was sobbing. Surrendering. To the one fate I was so sure I'd been assigned.

I waited for him to overtake me. His shame. His loneliness. His addiction. His trauma. His hopelessness.

But nothing came for me.

The world remained just as quiet as it had been before. My mind even more so. Even as tears streaked rivers from my bloodshot eyes and I let the long-repressed rage spill out, I was still me. Humbled. Stripped down. Weeping for what I'd lost. Childhood. Innocence.

Fuck. It wasn't my father's pain that awaited me in the corners of my heart that I hadn't dared to expose until now. It was the realization that underneath it all, I was still just a kid. A boy who'd done everything he could—gotten the grades, shown off his talents, kept the family secrets, made something of himself that most people dare not even dream of—had done *everything* in the hope that he'd prove himself worth staying for. Worth more than the demons his father carried, worth more than the whispers of his father's addiction.

I'd done everything in the hope that one day my father would sit me down, hold me close, and tell me that I could stop working so hard. That I didn't have to prove anything. That he loved me without conditions. That he'd always stay.

But everything I'd done hadn't been enough.

And it never will be.

He's never going to be what I wish he could be, is he?

That's the hard part about being anyone's child: parents can only be who they are. Sometimes who they are is what we want and need. Sometimes they can't even come close. But even as we grow into adults, we never stop wishing.

No, we don't.

I've spent my entire life trying to be more than him. To be everything he isn't. But it turns out that that's a fool's errand. How can I strive to be the things I've never seen? I don't know what healthy looks like. I don't know what manhood is. I don't know what fatherhood is supposed to be. All I know is what everything isn't.

I'm scared that I don't know how to be who I want to be.

Look, I know it's scary. And it feels like you've never had a hand to guide you. It's not fair and it sucks. But you know what? You're a fucking <u>doctor</u>. You know what healthy looks like. You've learned how to find it even when it's hidden beneath the nastiest, most life-threatening layers of bullshit.

I guess you're right, but—

And you're a <u>creative</u> doctor. I've watched you craft entire worlds out of your imagination. Weave stories and music and lives from next to nothing. All you've ever needed were whispers of inspiration.

I feel like all I've done with my imagination is weave stories about myself that have kept me trapped.

It was a way to survive. But now that the truth has been laid bare and you've bled all you can bleed, can you finally feel that living that way was a—

A choice.

Yes. A choice. So what will you choose now?

I'm not sure. But I'm awake. And my fingers are itching to write something new.

That sounds like a start.

Hey.

Thanks for coming back to me.

I was never truly gone. Just waiting. For you to stop being a dick.

I deserve that.

But seriously. You may get lonely, but I promise you'll never be alone.

Thank you. Now, if you'll excuse me, I have a letter to write.

To someone who's going to need reminding of how much his life is worth.

Anthony Lloyd Chin-Quee.

Junior.

Letter to a Young Bird

Good morning, young one
I've watched you
    Terrified to breathe
But in your first act of trust,
    pulling this world's air into your burning chest
To announce your arrival.
I looked into your eyes that instant
    and every moment since, young one.
I have seen your curiosity
I have seen your courage
I have seen your strength
I have seen your capacity for . . .
               (all things infinite)
And in your eyes, I have also seen understanding
that you too, just as I have,
have seen all of these things in yourself.
You have grown, young one.
And the world has grown with you.
The troubles have become more crucial
the universe has become far-reaching
ideas are everlasting
love is the ever-elusive magic—

you know it exists, you inhale it with each breath
you've been told it enfolds you
but you can't touch it.
you have never seen it.
and it rings false as soon as you speak its name
    the very mention tumbling the tower on which it
    was perched.
You look tired, young one.
    I see past the eyes that you put on display for the world.
They say that they've seen you fly.
But you and I know better.
You have floated.
You have coasted.
    and as magical as that may appear to untrained eyes
        you and I know that you were meant for more than this.
You were meant to soar.
This you have known since
that first magical eruption,
that first burning breath.
But your own expectations
    have made your wings heavy.
I have seen you look to the sky and wonder
        what are one bird's wing beats against the universe?
    What is one brilliant new flame in the world-sustaining light
    of the sun?
Yet today, in light of the dawn of your rebirth, I say to you that
the expectations
the fear
the doubt
the limits
    are of your own creation.
The weight of the world is an illusion.
It is your canvas
    paint it beautifully.

It is your opus
    add your grace notes.
Stare into the sun and shine as you were meant to.
It will not blind you
and your brilliance will not blind those who look to you
but will prism-break into every possibility they have ever known.
And even some that they haven't.
You were meant to fly.
And fly you will.
But then you will soar
into the everlasting expanse of your dreams.
Don't worry—
    you will breathe just fine up there
        and you will look into the sun with wide eyes.
And you will repeat to yourself every moment as you set your
    course ever upward:
My light was meant to shine.
My soul was born to fly.
And so it is.

SIX

RAINBOW CONNECTION

I've had the same anxiety dream for the last twenty years. I'm back in high school, and it's opening night of the play I'm in, and I don't know any of my lines or stage directions. I search frantically for my drama teacher so I can tell her that I'm unprepared and I shouldn't go on, but I can never find her. The curtain rises, the music plays, the audience gives an expectant round of applause, and I walk onstage. And before I can fake my way through my first line, I wake up.

I've had the dream twice this week—a pretty on-the-nose brain reaction as I prepare for my first formal public performance in years. I'd never reflected much on the deeper meaning of its recurrent presence in my brain until this morning. I got to thinking about fear, and how the deep ones find ways to invade and stay with you. They take root wherever you feel safest. Since my very first role as Lord Capulet in *Romeo and Juliet* at age ten, in those early moments of learning how completely I could create worlds to share with others, the stage was the place I always *wished* I could feel safe. But in truth, it was just a place where I could attempt honesty in disguise and convince myself that the audience could see the truth behind my borrowed words.

It was the closest thing to safe I had, so I tried my best to stretch the feeling as far as it would reach.

I've gone on to become an actor around family, friends, strangers, and acquaintances every day. Nobody but me knows that I walk through each day playing a role. Nobody knows the fear that bolsters my disguise. I thought acting could offer me protection from the dangers of the world and the uncontrollable feelings they'd awaken in me. But it hasn't worked the way I'd hoped.

I've walked through every day of my life that I haven't been onstage with a sickening pit of stage fright in my stomach. Afraid that the day would come where my preparation would slip, I'd forget all of my lines, and I'd expose the real me. And the world would hate it.

So I've been stuck. Wanting so badly for true sanctuary, terrified of the toll I'd have to pay for it.

Because the reality is that there is no safe haven when the world doesn't know who you really are.

The cute thing about babies is that they all have their own little personalities right out of the oven. And you should really pay attention to them, because those traits are usually the ones that they keep forever."

The spotlight was hot. A tingling current of vitality hummed through me, resulting in a curious degree of hypersensitivity: I could feel the ridges of creaking floorboards through my shoes, and each damp fiber of denim as I wiped sweaty palms on my jeans. I knew my lines and I knew my delivery—tell the story casually, as if it were an intimate conversation, and don't let them see just how much I'd practiced that relaxed familiarity. The audience was an expanse of murky darkness surrounding the halo of spotlight, but I knew the trick: to draw the entire audience in, focus my eyes on everybody and nobody. And don't forget to breathe.

"For me, I was a perfectionist. My mom always tells this story about how I started learning how to write really early because I wanted to be like the older kids, but my motor skills weren't passing muster. I practiced writing my name a little bit, but I just could not get three of the four letters to look right, so I ended up signing all of my finger-painting creations with nothing but a big letter *T*. *T* for Tony. I just refused to write any other letters until I knew I could do them perfectly. Pretty neurotic for a three-year-old, but that was me.

"Things got easier as I got older. School was always easy— learn the facts and you'll ace the test. But for high-stress human interactions, things got a little more complicated."

Suddenly, a handful of faces bloomed from the obscurity of the audience. Their features were hazy but undeniably familiar. Some grumbled in admonishing hushed tones to their neighbors. Others fixed me in their gazes, shaking their heads in warning.

Don't you do this . . . You know damn well you'll find no absolution here. Not among strangers.

It had to be my imagination. Had to be.

But real or not, they halted my performance in its tracks. For a moment, I couldn't remember why I was onstage in front of hundreds of people. I'd left my hospital after a twelve-hour shift and headed straight to a storytelling contest? That couldn't be right. That would be crazy. I should run.

My weight shifted as my legs itched for retreat. The wood panel creaked again beneath my big toe.

Hey. You're here. Be here. And don't forget—

To breathe.

"In the fall of my senior year of high school, I decided I had a crush on this girl from my theater class. I'd called her a few times, broken the ice, and eventually scored a big date on a Saturday afternoon. We were going to see some French medieval lamps or some similarly boring shit that she was into. They weren't exactly making history come alive, but hey, all in the name of adolescent love, right?

"So that morning I got fresh and headed downstairs to get my coat. I turned around to say goodbye to my mom. She was sitting at the kitchen table silhouetted in the sun. And she was shaking."

Without warning, I felt the electricity running through my skin shoot blazing sparks through my pores. A thousand tiny pinpricks. I couldn't stand still. I couldn't breathe through this. If I didn't move, if I didn't *run*, my crawling skin would leap clean off my body. A face in the second row let out a familiar chuckle that echoed between my ears for a moment. Then it whispered to me, the airy words reaching me as clearly as if its lips were brushing my ear.

Courage was never for you. And I will laugh and delight in watching your fragility shatter you as you find out why.

I knew that voice. The one that always found me just as I'd begun to fall. The one that had always been right. And this moment was no different.

Yes, I have been a coward. Courage was never for me.

Until now.

"She was looking down into her palms, and in each hand she

had a huge clump of hair. And she was crying so hard that she couldn't sit still. Because my mom had breast cancer. Chemotherapy was trying to kill it and strangling every other part of her body in the process. She never looked over at me.

"I zipped up my jacket, turned, and walked out of my front door without saying a word."

My voice echoed and died. And then silence, oppressive and disgusted. The faces of my detractors were impossible to identify. I was alone. Clothed only by shame and a corset of guilt, squeezing my chest until my ribs threatened to snap. I breathed in the quiet judgment of an audience held captive. It was thick and polluted, a fitting penance for my years of silence: asphyxiation by aerosolized contempt.

"And that's how I was when it came to my mom being sick and in pain. I was a ghost—I was never there for her. Intentionally. The idea of trying to be there and not knowing if I could do it 'correctly' was paralyzing. So instead I was just . . . never there at all."

More silence. Then that same voice. Closer now. Louder. Filling my mind with a derisive hiss.

You stay right there. Don't say another word. Feel this weight. This is what you've always deserved.

Yes. The moment was long overdue.

"Eventually she beat the cancer, life went on, and even though she always told me that she was never disappointed in me, I never was able to forgive myself for those days. I mean, what kind of son, no matter how teenage and emo he was, made himself scarce while his mom was fighting for her life?"

You! shouted a thundering voice.

Was it them? Was it me? Was there a difference anymore?

"And of course," I continued through a clenched jaw, "I ended up going on to repeat that pattern in one way or another over the years. Sabotaging myself professionally, sabotaging relationships—all because I felt the world getting too large, too difficult to control and do well."

My jaw muscles loosened slightly. "Then, two months ago, I got a phone call from my mom telling me that after fourteen years, she'd just found out that her breast cancer had come back. And I knew in my heart that the universe was shaking me awake and telling me that this time, everything had to be different."

I could see that night as clearly as I remembered the day I'd walked out on her. I'd been back at work in the hospital for just a few weeks after my forced leave of absence. I'd passed Step 3 the second time I took the test and matriculated into my third year of residency. The demands on my knowledge and time and skills had multiplied. But where I'd allowed them to pull me apart just weeks before, I'd committed on the flight back from Mexico to take control. No more reacting to a life that happened to me. My approaches and responses to the daily challenges were mine to craft. It would just take practice. After all, I was unlearning a lifetime of bad habits. So every day would be an exercise in self-preservation—making routines, asking for help, expressing gratitude, fulfilling small daily promises to myself, all so that I could make survival palatable, achievable.

And then the surprise conference call between me, my mom, and my two younger brothers that threatened to capsize my efforts. Cancer. Again. She was scared—I could hear it in the way she tried to recite the memorized words of explanation. My brothers were scared too: they were betrayed by their silence.

Me? I remember a voice in my head informing me that it was time to be afraid. I'd replied, *Yes, it is. But this time, we stay.*

The memory of that night splashed over me like ice water. The audience came into sharper focus. Shadowed faces of strangers, attentive and expectant. The familiar voices, the murmurs of judgment, were gone.

I was present.

This time we stay.

"So, I knew that the plan was for her to have an enormous, very risky and dangerous surgery—twelve hours long with two surgical teams. And since I'm her doctor son, I spoke with her two surgeons every other day for a month and a half so that I knew every detail of the plan. It was completely terrifying to me, but I broke it down for my mom so that she understood and could ask the right questions.

"Information was one thing, but more importantly, I'd be damned if she'd feel alone or unsupported by me this time around. So one day I woke up with an idea: I sent an email to all of my closest friends from over the years, and the message was very simple: My mom's cancer had come back, and I was half a country away from her while she was using all of her own strength just to wake up every morning. I'd recently learned that in this life sometimes you've got to give up this idea of trying to take control of everything. Sometimes you've got to trust the hands that enfold you to lift you up. So please, lift her up.

"I got over twenty responses and they were overwhelming, ranging from hilarious anecdotes to Bible verses to poetry. And every other day I'd choose one and send it to her. And all she could ever tell me was that they were always on time. Through these she was reminded not only of how much she was cared for but of just how much her lessons and her love had spread to people all over the country through me and how I'd lived my life. And I think they lit up some of her darkest days."

I found myself smiling as I rode the story's momentum of love and fear. The theater felt warmer. My voice barely echoed, as it was being absorbed by a few hundred souls' rapt attention. I wasn't alone anymore.

I was safe.

I was home.

"Before I knew it, it was the morning of surgery. We had seen the doctors, the nurses had placed IVs, and for a moment it was just the two of us. She sat up in her bed, and she was shaking."

Can I truly—

Keep going.

"The first tears fell down her cheeks."

This time—

I stay.

"And there was not one bone in my body that wanted to run away. I wrapped both of my arms around her, and all she could get out was that she was 'so scared . . . and it's gonna be okay, right? Everything's going to be okay? What happens to you and your brothers if . . . What if this is it? What if this is the end?'"

The words that my mother believed could be her last hung in the stillness of the dark theater, kept aloft by the determined baritone of her eldest son. And just as they did when I first heard them at her bedside, they robbed me of the last of my strength.

I reached a hand for the microphone and held on tight.

"I don't know if anyone here has looked their parent in the eyes in a moment when they think they're going to die."

And just then, something unseen propped me up.

"All I could think to say was 'Guess what? You have a lot more work to do. But for today, let the rest of us do the work.'"

I lifted my head higher. My voice, now fully supported for the first time all night, found the balcony with ease.

"And then it was time. In a flurry of curtains, nurses, and squeaky bed wheels, she was rolling toward the operating room doors. And I didn't realize it at the time, but as she rolled away I was singing this song that always reminded me of her—from *The Muppet Movie*, of all things.

"You know, the one that goes: 'Someday we'll find it, the rainbow connection / The lovers, the dreamers and me . . .'"

I hadn't always understood what Kermit was talking about. The melody and amphibian soul behind the banjo had always been enough to set my mind adrift independent of the lyrics. I didn't understand it the day of my mother's surgery—it had just managed to find me. But that night onstage, I found it. The rainbow connection. It was a bridge back to the world beyond myself. It led to a land where the intangible unseen was just as important a part of me as the world I could touch and feel. There was courage in love. There was strength in dreams. And the divine? Well . . .

"And then she was gone. For fourteen hours. She woke up at the end to her three sons at her bedside. All of the cancer was out, and she wouldn't need more chemo. I asked her a few days later if she felt that I'd been there this time around.

"Her smile faded then. Her eyes bored into mine for an interminable moment. Then she spoke slowly, so that I might at long last understand: 'Please forgive yourself. I am so proud of you.'

"So I guess what I'd say to everyone here is . . ."

I paused, recognizing a persistent, albeit newly weak voice in my head. It whispered a strained, airy plea.

Please get this right. You have to get this last part right.

I smiled. It would take years of daily practice to unlearn this reflex, but here's where I'd start.

I was going to give it to the world. Whether it was right or not.

"I'd say go ahead and sign your whole name to your finger-painting masterpieces. The letters may be shaky, but it will without a doubt find its way onto the refrigerator door, held fast with a gold-star magnet. Because your best will always be good enough."

Just then, I recognized the magic in the air around me, transforming my posture into a stance of pride, carrying my voice on its wings, holding my eyes wide to receive all of the light they had been missing. I sensed that it had followed me around for a long time, just out of sight. It had been present in all of my choices; in the moments I'd stubbornly clung to life through the pain; in the ways that I trusted and had been trusted; the ways in which I'd created and been created; the ways I'd loved and been loved. The magic had always been surrounding and within me. Every day. All I'd ever needed to do was greet it. And let it out.

And for the first time, I realized that this magic had a name. One that I'd spent decades searching for, hoping to believe in even after I'd convinced myself that I'd given up.

Hi, God.

I'm sorry for abandoning you.

Thank you for never abandoning me.

As if in joyful response to our reunion, the magic offered a warm embrace through my final words to the audience of strangers.

"Your best will probably be someone else's perfect."

SEVEN

Y'AIN'T (K)NO(W)

O kay, so when do you want to take it out?" I asked as I rounded
a corner, entering the overnight observation wing.

Pale morning light crept through the window at the end of the
corridor. At 6:50 a.m. on a Saturday, the hallway was buzzing with
activity—pagers blared from every corner, nurses gave morning
reports to each other in pairs along the wall, and heart monitors
chirped from within dark patient rooms.

To my right was the weekend ENT attending, Dr. Krohn, a
study in the art of appearing chronically unimpressed. Behind us
strode two junior residents—Liam, phone glued to his ear as he
scrawled notes into the corner of an already crowded page, and
Jazlyn, struggling to tame her messy bun of hair with a tie as she
trotted quickly to my side to answer the question.

Because I got to be the one who asked some of the questions
these days. A perk of being a fourth-year resident. A *senior* resident. It was now my job to lead morning rounds, keep them organized and efficient, and, of course, make my junior residents look

good to the boss even as they struggled to keep their heads above water.

That last part wasn't an official requirement, and definitely hadn't been a grace that had been extended to me very often over the last few years, but I was determined to try out a groundbreaking approach to residency training: don't be a full-time asshole.

"Well, he's post-op day one," replied Jazlyn. "No anticoagulation, and the gauze was only placed as a precaution, so I'd say it could come out . . . tonight?"

I stole a glance at Dr. Krohn as he raised an eyebrow at Jazlyn's response, immediately making him appear even more unimpressed. Jazlyn swore under her breath as she ducked quickly behind me to avoid an oncoming recklessly driven stretcher.

"It *could* come out tonight," I said over my shoulder, "but do you see any potential issues with that plan?"

I could almost hear the wheels turning in Jazlyn's head. She ventured a hesitant ". . . Yes?"

"Such as?"

"Well," she said, reaching frantically for an answer she wasn't sure of. The life of a junior resident in a nutshell. "He could bleed if I take it out? But that's always a risk, right?"

I threw her a bone. "And do you look forward to taking that risk on a Saturday night, when the nurses tend to be less comfortable with these types of patients and will thus be calling you every hour to ask if every drop of pink spit that comes out of his trach tube is a bloody emergency?"

"Not really."

"So?"

Jazlyn smiled, finally seeing the solution. "I'll take it out tomorrow morning when I know the A team is around?"

"Very nice," muttered Dr. Krohn. I offered her a *good job* nod. She threw back an *I'm brilliant no big deal* shrug.

Kids today. No respect.

"Okay, who's next?" Dr. Krohn muttered through sallow jowls. He looked expectantly at me. I looked to Jazlyn, who was scribbling a quick note on her patient list. Recognizing the silence, she looked up, the panic of the hot seat in her eyes. I cocked my head and felt a hint of a smile creep into my lips.

You may be brilliant, but you're not out of the woods yet, I thought. *Show us what else you've got.*

"Sorry! Sorry, Dr. Krohn. Um, this next patient . . ." Jazlyn shuffled through the loose pages of notes she'd pulled from her pocket. "So, this is Kevon Harris, nineteen-year-old male, who presented with a complaint of sore throat for the last two weeks that suddenly got worse yesterday, resulting in difficulty swallowing and lots of drooling. Exam was consistent with peritonsillar abscess on the left, which I attempted to drain, however I didn't pull back any fluid. So I started him on clindamycin and dexamethasone and admitted him for observation until he can tolerate drinking liquids."

Dr. Krohn puffed out his chest. "Well," he proclaimed, projecting clearly for the first time that morning, "seems like as good a time as any for a little anatomy quiz."

The impromptu Socratic questioning session, aka every junior resident's nightmare. Jazlyn visibly deflated. I was going to have to work with her on her poker face.

"Dr. Bacani," continued Dr. Krohn, his eyes boring into Jazlyn, "what are the five arteries that supply the tonsils?"

"Well"—her eyes shot back and forth across the linoleum floor tiles—"there are the ascending and descending palatine, the dorsal lingual, the tonsillar branch of the facial artery . . ."

Shit. She was stuck. She withered under Dr. Krohn's self-important smirk until he turned his gaze to Liam, who'd been following the proceedings silently.

"Dr. O'Connell?"

"The ascending pharyngeal artery from the internal carotid," Liam said quickly. He'd been locked and loaded.

"Very nice, Liam."

It struck me that there was no way for Dr. Krohn to have known that Liam knew all of the other arteries. He could have just gotten lucky that Jazlyn had done the hard part. Nonetheless, Liam got the kudos and Jazlyn winced as if stricken.

"So, Dr. Bacani," continued Dr. Krohn, now relishing his time in the spotlight, "we'll give you another chance. Did you get a CT scan for this patient?"

"No, sir," Jazlyn replied confidently.

"And why is that?"

"Because peritonsillar abscess is a clinical diagnosis. I felt my physical exam was sufficient."

She was right.

"Interesting. And would you agree with that, Liam?"

"I would," said Liam, a bit less confident than he'd been a minute before.

Dr. Krohn smirked, puffed out his chest once again, and turned to me. I studied him, unsure what he was playing at.

"And how about our senior resident? Would you venture a different answer?"

"No," I replied. Dr. Krohn stood up a bit taller, clearly preparing to hold court with a lengthy "teachable moment" when I went on, "I think the real question we're circling here is whether or not getting a CT scan would change our management. And I don't believe that it would."

The two junior residents held their breath as Dr. Krohn silently appraised me.

"Really?" said Dr. Krohn. "And what if he's got an abscess that was missed by Dr. Bacani's drainage attempt? A CT would show that. Wouldn't you like to know if that were the case?"

"I don't think I would." I could see where Dr. Krohn was trying to lead us, but he was wrong. I knew it, as did Jazlyn and Liam. I'd been studying and treating these types of abscesses daily for four years. The management plan was clear. I didn't know what Dr. Krohn's motivations were for confusing the juniors, but it was time to step up and look after them.

I went on, "First of all, I'm confident in Dr. Bacani's ability to perform an adequate exam and PTA drainage. Second, CT scans aren't great at telling the difference between early abscess formation and localized infectious inflammation. Regardless of what we might see, we would watch the patient's clinical exam. If he's getting better on the medications, then he doesn't need a scan."

"Let me phrase this differently." Dr. Krohn was breathing heavily now, doing his best to appear in charge and menacing. "I want you to get a CT scan for this patient."

"But can I ask why?"

He stepped closer to me and responded with strained, measured calm, "Because I would like to know if the patient has an abscess."

Dr. Krohn was known among the residents for this type of bullying fuckery. As far as he was concerned, the hierarchy of power in the hospital was to be respected at all costs and never to be questioned, because he believed he'd forgotten more ENT information than we'd ever learn.

But fuck that. He was wrong. What had I been studying all these years for, if not to be able to distinguish fact from fiction?

"And if the scan definitively shows an abscess, that would force our hand to perform another drainage today, which he may not even need. Because the antibiotics and steroids are likely already treating him."

Dr. Krohn's nostrils flared. His chest heaved. Rage simmered just beneath his skin in his tensed muscles and rabid, wild stare.

I didn't flinch.

"What I'd recommend is observation today," I continued, standing tall. "We give him a chance to feel better. If he can eat and drink by the morning, we send him home. If nothing's changed by tomorrow, or he takes a dive and gets worse later today, we'll scan him. I just feel like if we can safely spare him the costs of an unnecessary scan, then—"

"*Enough!*"

All movement in the corridor came to a momentary halt as my extremely professional boss roared at the top of his lungs inches from my face—in a fucking hospital. I could sense the junior residents going rigid beside me. He must have seen that my expression was not one of fear but more in the neighborhood of *is this motherfucker kidding me*, because he quickly closed the gap between us and brought his lips uncomfortably close to my ears.

"You're on thin fucking ice."

He stepped back and composed himself, took a quick look at the junior residents, who were making themselves busy with whatever paperwork they could get their hands on, then turned back to me, looking me in the eyes for what would be the last time that morning.

"You need to learn some fucking respect," he spat, spinning on his heel and disappearing into the patient room. Jazlyn and Liam scurried after him, heads down.

I stayed in the hallway, feet rooted to the linoleum, and breathed. Slowly, in and out, willing my jaw muscles to relax and my fists to unclench. It was a practiced form of instant meditation, and one I'd been using often at the hospital this past year whenever I'd suffer public indignities. But this time? Holy shit, was it hard.

Bro. Listen. You know I generally subscribe to nonviolence. But when I tell you I would have given you a pass . . .

Yo, you know how aggressively I suppress my hoodstincts[1] every fucking day in order to stay employed, alive, and out of jail, but that motherfucker right there nearly made me risk it all.

I mean, I'm happy to fantasize with you till the cows come home about backhanding your boss and stomping him the fuck out, but you know me—I'm the question guy. So I've got to ask: After all of the fucked-up moments, all of the disrespectful jokes and backhanded compliments and dressings-down you've endured over the last four years, what made this one different? Why'd this one leave you—

Shivering with rage in a hospital hallway?

I think it's because I knew in an instant that, without question (and that's a big deal, because I always question my judgment and sanity when I feel myself on the edge of an outsize reaction), he would never have spoken to my coresident Peyton that way.

---

1. Hoodstincts = hood instincts, aka the primal urge to let a motherfucker know (by any means necessary) that disrespect will not be tolerated. Means may include verbal lashings, engagement in psychological warfare, and the throwing of all manner of hands. Of note: one need not have originated in the hood to harbor hoodstincts.

And the main difference between Peyton and me?

Mm-hmm. Why don't you take me back to the moment you met the ENT department's favorite white boy?

*I*rregardless is not a word.

Despite that, my fucking spell-check says that it actually is.

The dictionary definition of *irregardless* is *regardless*: you know—the *actual* word people mean to say. Farther down the page, the descendants of George and Charles Merriam and Noah Webster (as well as the residents of the newest part of Oxford) wrote in an important note on the word's usage—something to the effect of "Fine, we'll recognize *irregardless* as a word since dumb people have been conflating *irrespective* and *regardless* for so long that we're powerless to stop it . . . but please, don't say it if you're trying to sound smart or professional."

I love intelligence. And language. And words.

So I fucking hate when people say "irregardless." If I find myself in conversation with someone who favors its usage, it's typically grounds for dismissal from my pending offer of friendship or respect.

And of course, it was one of the first one hundred words I heard fall out of my coresident's mouth on the day we first met four years ago.

Still, I liked the guy.

Maybe it's because Peyton looked so . . . we'll say sturdy. Thick neck, short-cropped chestnut hair, broad shoulders, and a military posture that added a couple more inches to his already impressive height. As corn-fed as the cow that had been slaughtered to make the cheeseburger he'd just devoured. The kid was definitely built to last. And even under the tired pub lighting in our corner booth, I could see in his eyes that his body wasn't the only thing forged in the unforgiving Rust Belt of the Midwest. He was a workhorse. Tireless. A willing soldier. Eager to please. He might not always be the smartest guy in the room, but damn it, he was going to succeed *irregardless*. It was admittedly charming. I cracked a grin as I dipped another chicken finger in some good-ass sauce.

And oh boy, was he ever a fan of Chin-Quee. I was from Brooklyn! That's so cool! And I went to Harvard! He'd never met anyone who'd gone there before! Weren't they all supergeniuses there?! I seemed so normal! Did I really beatbox heart murmurs during my residency interview?! No way, that's incredible! He couldn't believe it when he first heard the rumor, but now that he'd met me he totally got it! Was I into movies?! How about TV shows?! Had I seen this show called *Black-ish*?! He and his wife love it!

Peyton was starstruck. By *me*. The coolest person he'd ever met in his life, and he was completely sure of it within minutes of breaking bread with me for the first time. This sort of lavish, immediate praise and validation might have bolstered the ego of one less skeptical and world-weary, but (surprise) that's not me. My honorary degree in Caucasoid studies had given me the tools to lift his effusive reaction to my existence off our table and place it in a file full of a life's worth of similar experiences.

Of course I was the coolest person he'd ever met in his life. Because I'm Black. Well-meaning white people have heard all their lives about how cool we are, but most observe it from a distance. Peyton had a front-row seat to the show for the first time, and he was hoping to be wowed. And holy cow, he'd never imagined that he'd find himself in proximity to a dude who not only checked all of the cool-Black-guy boxes but also had already achieved levels of success beyond anything anyone in his world had ever dreamed. My life was exotic. A once-in-a-lifetime, can't-miss attraction. I was so incredible that he couldn't even summon the postgraduation med student default sentiments of jealousy and competitiveness. I was a newly discovered animal on display at the zoo. He couldn't envy or resent the otherworldly colors of my plumage or the power coiled in my every graceful step, because I was a *completely different species*. He'd stare slack-jawed at me through the glass and then hurry home to try to capture the wonderment in words for his family and friends.

I took another bite of breaded chicken and sat back, unable to begrudge him his perceptions. My confidence in white folks' ability to ask themselves critical questions about their whiteness has never been very high, so I let Peyton continue living his joyful reverie. His blue eyes sparkled when he leaned in and spoke in an earnest, hushed tone.

"I'm so glad that we're going to get to work together. I think we're going to be really great friends."

Sure. Why not?

After all, my assessment was complete: Peyton was harmless. I smiled ruefully down at my empty plate as the repercussions of his "good guy" persona fell like dominoes through my head. His harmlessness would prove the most harmful thing about him. Harmless people don't rock the boat. They aren't loud, they aren't courageous, and when push came to shove (and I had an inkling that our upcoming years of residency training would shove far more often than not), he wouldn't choose me. He'd choose harmless.

I'd had plenty of harmless white friends in my life. Very good at cheerleading. And even better at disappearing when life got uncomfortable.

And I'd been content to let them, their world, their whiteness, wash over me as one of the most basic facts of life. Their love was fickle, their temperaments childish and self-serving, and their power absolute—ingrained in the fabric of this country. Of this world, really. So my life was at their mercy. I could either ride the wave or drown.

But now?

Now, in this moment, as I think about all of the Peytons I've be-friended and all of the Dr. Krohns I've appeased in the last thirty years, I'm fucking *furious*. Like, deeply, soul-shakingly incensed. And this brand of anger feels different than it ever has in the past. I used to be able to brush it off and let it go, because what was the point in staying mad when I was dealing with the thoughtless and careless actions of people who continually demonstrated how little I mattered to them? Fuck them. I'd find a way to succeed regardless.

But now, as I still tremble from that moment on rounds, I can't shake the feeling that it's been so much more than carelessness. I'm pretty sure that they do care about me. A lot. They care about what my life and success mean for them. What it might mean to others who look like me or have lived like me.

They care so much about me that they're terrified of me.

They care enough about me to hate me.

And they hate me enough to want me gone. Destroyed.

They hate me enough to want me dead.

And I think they've actually been trying to kill me for a very, very long time.

But you're still not 100 percent sure.

I mean, how can I be? I'm basically flirting with upending my entire worldview here. I don't know if I'm ready to do that. Plus, I'm still simmering. Maybe my anger is clouding my perspective? Exaggerating, conflating, and confusing some things?

Maybe anger, or rather the recognition that your anger is warranted and has been simmering far longer and more consistently than you've wanted to accept, is exactly what you need in order to know with certainty that you're right.

Shit. Maybe it's time to look back at some of the moments that made me. New perspective. New lens.

You were too close, too in the moment when you experienced them the first go-round. Try sitting in the audience this time.

I mean, it has been awhile since I've watched a good movie.

You Want Your Favorite Negro Dead

Lived in and Directed by:
Your Boy C-Q

FADE IN:

INT. PUBLIC SCHOOL AUDITORIUM—1994—MORNING

Applause booms as a small chorus of 10-year-olds sings
the last note of an inspirational pop song. The place
is packed. Standing room only. Smartly dressed children
fill the front half of the seats while proud parents
jockey for photo-op positions in the back.

A banner hangs over the stage: <u>CONGRATULATIONS 5TH</u>
<u>GRADE GRADUATES!</u>

We close in on two suited boys: my friend DAVID leans
over to ME (10 years old), clip-on tie in hand.

>   DAVID
> Are you gonna make a speech?

>   ME
> I think I'm just supposed to take the
> certificate and go.

>   DAVID
> Oh man, that's boring. Grab the mic and
> yell, "School sucks!" I totally dare
> you.

I smile, shake my head, and turn to scan the crowd. MY
MOTHER waves animatedly and shoots out of her chair to
snap a picture, shaking off MY FATHER's embarrassed grip.

A hush falls over the crowd as the principal, MR. LEVITAN,
takes to the stage and holds two fingers in the air. The
children follow suit in silence. Well trained.

                    MR. LEVITAN
          Good morning, boys and girls.

                    ALL OF THE KIDS
                    (in unison)
          Good morning, Mr. Levitan!

                    MR. LEVITAN
          Graduating students, parents, we've
          come to the final honor of our
          ceremony: the class valedictorian.
          The student with the highest record
          of academic achievement in the entire
          school.

David taps me excitedly with his clip-on tie. I shift
restlessly in my seat.

                    MR. LEVITAN
          The valedictorian of this year's
          class . . .

My Mother jostles for position in the gaggle of chitter-
ing parents.

                    MR. LEVITAN
          Jason Finklestein!

Applause explodes around me. JASON makes his way down the
row past my knees. David sits stunned.

                    DAVID
          What the heck? Everyone knows you have
          the best grades!

I turn to my parents, who are engaged in several furrowed-brow conversations with their neighbors. Emotions I can't read from my seat.

Not everyone is clapping.

I turn back to my friend.

> ME
>
> Maybe I didn't.

I look to the stage and join in the applause as Jason receives my school's highest honor.

CUT TO:

INT. CHIN-QUEE HOUSEHOLD—MID-1990S—AFTERNOON

A TV sits on a forest-green shag carpet. A busty supermodel-turned-actress pouts through the screen, scantily clad, gun in hand. On a couch a few feet away sit MY FATHER and ME (12-ish years old), eyes glued to the idiot box.

> ME
>
> So why can't I marry a white girl?

> MY FATHER
> (eyes on the screen)
>
> Hmm?

> ME
>
> You used to tell me that all the time when I was little but, like, they're cool. They're in my classes. Some of them are my friends. They're as nice as anyone else.

My Father chuckles at that, then squints his eyes at the
white woman filling the screen.

> MY FATHER
>> They can be your friends. But you
>> can't trust them. Because they'll never
>> understand you.

My face twists with a hundred retorts and a thousand
questions, but before I can speak—

> MY FATHER
>> Think of it this way: white girls are
>> for practice. Have your fun, figure
>> yourself out. They're great for that.
>> Just don't bring them home.

I turn back to the TV. Frustrated and unsatisfied. Silence
for a moment as the show returns from commercial break.

> MY FATHER
>> Actually, if you must bring one home,
>> make sure she looks like that.

We take a second to ogle the bouncing, gunslinging beauty
on the screen.

> MY FATHER
>> Plain Jane white girls are just the
>> worst. But with one of these, at least
>> we'll have something to look at!

My Father smiles. I nod in contemplation of the day's
sermon.

CUT TO:

EXT. BROOKLYN STREET CORNER—LATE 1990S—NIGHT

Three bubble jackets. Three beanie hats. Three puffs of frozen air escaping the mouths of three Black men in training: SHEA, THOMAS, and ME (all of us 16-ish).

Rush hour rages on Flatbush Avenue as the city freezes with the setting of the sun. Shea and I huddle under the awning of a travel agency. Thomas holds one hand in the air at the curb, hoping to hail a cab, then retreats toward us, hopping to keep warm.

                    THOMAS
          Yo, I think it's time to just
          take the bus.

                    SHEA
          We wouldn't have made it in time on
          the bus twenty minutes ago, and we
          damn sure ain't making it now.

                    THOMAS
          Fuck, my dude. Going to see *Fight Club*
          is the only thing that got me through
          this week.

                    ME
          We'll make it. Who's up? Me? I'm
          feeling lucky this time.

JINGLING from a nearby door. The boys turn to see a middle-aged WHITE LADY poke her head out of the travel agency entrance.

                    WHITE LADY
          Hey!

                         SHEA
          Sorry, miss, we can move away from
          your window.

                     WHITE LADY
          No, no that's not . . . I've just been
          watching you guys for the last half
          hour and . . . Do you need some help?

                          ME
          No, we're fine. Just busy out here, you
          know? Rush hour.

She studies us for a moment, then ducks back inside. I
jog over to the curb and hold my hand out.

                         SHEA
          So is it, like, based on a true story?
          Like, do white people get together
          for book clubs and then just start
          slapping the shit out of each other?

                       THOMAS
          No, ass. The shit is a high-concept
          existential drama.

JINGLING. The White Lady emerges fully this time, bundled
in her coat and scarf, and jogs to the curb. She stops
a few feet in front of me and sticks out her arm. My
mouth drops in shock. I turn to my friends. Shea mouths
an indignant *"The fuck?"*

A cab pulls over in front of the White Lady in seconds.
She opens the rear door, turns to me.

                     WHITE LADY
          You guys better get in.

Shea and Thomas jog over. The White Lady steps aside to let me in, and the cab JERKS forward, nearly throwing me into the street. The White Lady springs to the passenger door and SLAMS the roof with both hands.

> WHITE LADY
> (at the cabbie)
> Hey! They are getting in this car! My
> God, you should be ashamed of yourself!

We clamber into the back seat. She closes the door behind us. A nod and a smile before she heads back to her office. The yellow cab pulls into rush hour traffic.

Three boys watch the streetlights pass in silence, shoulders drooped just a bit lower than they were five minutes prior.

CUT TO:

CLOSE-UP OF A TELEVISION SCREEN

Through sporadic bands of VHS distortion we see a pair of legs in khaki pants bouncing restlessly beneath a classroom desk. The image pans up slowly, revealing a bit more of this young student; hands clasped on the desk, sweater-vest and oversize T-shirt draping a bony frame, and a face—ME (17-ish years old), staring intently at my hands.

A chyron at the bottom of the screen reads: STUDENT DIVERSITY ROUNDTABLE.

I look up at the CAMERA.

> ME
> You sure you want me to answer that?

Nervous chuckles from off-screen. I crack a smile and nod.

                    ME
         Do I think that racism has affected my
         experience at this school? Absolutely.

The camera zooms out slowly, revealing a circle of students in a classroom: 90 percent white kids.

                    ME
         I'm not sure you guys know how much
         your education costs, but it's about
         sixteen thousand dollars a year to
         attend this school.

Slowly we ZOOM OUT from the TELEVISION SCREEN to find that it sits on a rolling stand on the stage of a—

INT. CHAPEL-STYLE AUDITORIUM—PRIVATE SCHOOL—YEAR 2000—DAY

The place reeks of old money: sculpted pillars, stained glass, vaulted ceiling. My voice reverberates from the TV into the massive space.

               ME (ON TV)
         My family could never afford to send
         me here without help, so I'm on about
         ninety-eight percent financial aid.
         I've been told that I maintain it
         through my academic performance, but I
         know there's more to it than that.

We continue to ZOOM OUT and find pews full to bursting with students. Demographics are unsurprising: 250 teenage white faces, 16 in shades of brown. All eyes on the TV screen.

                         ME (ON TV)

          Not only am I smart, but I'm not
          threatening. Always smiling. I don't
          play sports; I act and choreograph
          dance and play music. I've been on
          panels at countless info sessions for
          potential new students and their
          families because I "make this community
          stronger." And I know this is because I
          am the right kind of Black student.

Restless murmurs rumble among the white students.

                         ME (ON TV)

          But you know who wasn't the right kind
          of Black? My little brother who had
          the audacity to get the same average
          grades that his white friends received.
          Or my cousin: arguably a genius, but
          too gay to be shown off in the
          promotional materials.

The Black students nod silently. They all remember.

                         ME (ON TV)

          Mysteriously, our school was unable to
          find the money to continue their
          financial aid, and thus I'm the only
          member of my family still here. But
          even now, I appreciate the clarity of
          the message they sent to us: if you're
          not our token Black student, we don't
          want you.

In the sea of gobsmacked white faces, we finally find
ME, watching myself on-screen with all the others. My
gaze shifts to meet the eyes of MR. FREEMAN, the balding

Caucasian headmaster (problematic private school-speak for principal). He stands at a podium on one side of the stage, expressionless but red in the face.

>   ME (ON TV)
>   So yes, racism has affected my
>   experience at this school. And it's
>   affected yours. You just never had to
>   pay attention.

I don't flinch under Mr. Freeman's boiling gaze. The video on the TV screen flickers and turns to static.

All eyes turn to Mr. Freeman.

His eyes hold the fear of a caged beast. Momentarily, he'll summon me to—

INT. HEADMASTER'S OFFICE—PRIVATE SCHOOL—MINUTES LATER

Mr. Freeman studies me from a seat behind a giant mahogany desk. Calculating.

>   MR. FREEMAN
>   Well, quite a morning!

My silence unnerves him. Spurs him on.

>   MR. FREEMAN
>   Listen, Tony. I think there's been a
>   misunderstanding.

>   ME
>   I really don't think there has.

>   MR. FREEMAN
>   I can assure you that there are not,
>   nor have there ever been, any

race-based practices involved in our
distribution of financial aid.

>   ME
> Fine then, assure me. I would love to
> hear your explanation of what happened
> to my family.

>   MR. FREEMAN
>   (bristling)
> It's . . . it's complicated.

I shake my head. *He's got to do better than that, and he knows it.*

Mr. Freeman shifts slightly in his seat. I lean forward, eager to see which path he chooses.

>   MR. FREEMAN
> What can I do to resolve this?

I smile. *Coward.*

>   ME
> You mean what can you do to make this
> go away? Nothing. After today you're
> going to have to start answering a lot
> of uncomfortable questions, and I'm not
> going to help you do it.

Mr. Freeman's locked jaw muscles pulse beneath his skin.

>   ME
> What can you do to make it up to my
> family? Nothing. They've moved on and
> never want to do business with you
> again. But you feel guilty. You want to

do something so badly. So it will have
to be for me.

I lean back, cross my legs, completely in control.

                    ME
          I'll make it easy for you. I'm
          submitting my application to Harvard
          in a couple of weeks. I want you to
          write a glowing, personalized letter of
          recommendation for me. My academic
          prowess, my diverse talents. My courage
          to speak up against injustices.

Mr. Freeman winces at that.

                    ME
          Honestly, I know I can get in without
          your help. But this would just be
          icing on the cake. Thoughts?

I raise my eyebrows as the headmaster realizes he's been
bested by a teenager. All before the third-period
bell.

                                        CUT TO:

EXT. OUTDOOR TENNIS COURT—EARLY AUGHTS—DAY

POP. A Serena-esque GRUNT. A yellow ball skips off a
white line. A racquet swings for it. Misses
terribly.

A body collapses to the ground, laughing in exhaustion:
ME (19-ish, ambitious wisps of facial hair on my chin).
I look up at my ragtag group of doubles players, Black
men all: on the opposing side of the net JERMAINE and
OBI share a high five; SAMMIE stands over me.

                    SAMMIE
Chin-Quee, you gotta get there!
Backhand, dude, backhand!

                     ME
               (gasping for air)
You told me this was like big
Ping-Pong. This is not big Ping-Pong!

                  JERMAINE
Okay, I'm willing to enact the mercy
rule. This is getting tragic.

                     OBI
Yeah, go get you a cool drink, and a
wheelchair.

                     ME
               (getting up slowly)
Nope. It's spring break and I'm here to
flex on you hoes. Big Ping-Pong,
motherfucker! Run it back!

The boys erupt in laughter, continuing to rib one another
as two OLDER WHITE MEN in their sixties approach from the
neighboring court.

                 WHITE MAN #1
     Hey!

Our laughter is cut short.

                    SAMMIE
     Hey, what's up?

                        WHITE MAN #1
            Time's up on this court.

                           JERMAINE
            I'm sorry?

                        WHITE MAN #2
            It's reserved.

                              ME
            Sorry, sir, but that's not how it
            works. This is a public court. I
            checked with the park manager. First
            come, first served.

                        WHITE MAN #1
            You boys must be visiting from out of
            town, so I'll make it clear: we have
            this court reserved. Your time is up.

A standoff. Tension hangs in the silence. I'm about to
take a step closer to the two men when—

                           JERMAINE
            All right, gentlemen, you win. We'll
            pack it up—

                              ME
            Sir, what is your plan exactly? You two
            going to stretch out over two courts?
            Because I don't think that's how the
            game is played.

Sammie puts a hand on my arm. I shake it off.

                                    ME

          No! No, this is bullshit. We're going
          to play right here on this court until
          we're done. If you two want to call
          the manager over, be my fucking guest.

The two white men smirk at me, as if I've just given them
a gift. White Man #1 pulls out his phone. Jermaine grabs
me by the shoulders and walks me off the court.

                                JERMAINE

          We're going.

                                    ME

          Come on, man, this is—

                                JERMAINE

          Tony. This is Florida. We're really far
          from home. You understand what I'm
          saying?

Jermaine takes my racquet and slips it into a bag, his
eyes never leaving mine. He nods at me. Pleading.

                                    ME

          Yeah.

I didn't understand. But I left the court all the same.

                                                      CUT TO:

INT. ANOTHER HEADMASTER'S OFFICE—2006—DAY

ME again. 22 years old. Goatee. Shirt and tie.
Shoulders slumped. Eyes downcast. Barely sitting
upright in an armchair across from BILL PEMBERTON—a
kindly, wrinkled 60-year-old white man in the
headmaster's seat.

                              BILL
          Well, I'll admit this is a sad
          surprise. In the year you've been
          here, you've been a tremendous asset
          to our faculty. The students rave
          about you; feedback from the parents
          has been excellent. But in the
          interest of our continued growth as a
          community, may I ask why you feel you
          need to leave?

My eyes lift slowly. They are hollow, lifeless. Desperate. A mirthless chuckle escapes my lips.

                              ME
          I should have known. I should have
          known when you fuckers told me that I
          was one of two new Black teachers—the
          first Black teachers in this school's
          one-hundred-forty-year history. I
          should have known that I was more
          "board mandate" than "legitimate
          candidate."

I stand, stroll to a bookcase, thumb through volumes.

                              ME
          But your other teachers sure as hell
          knew. And I'm sure they thought I'd be
          harmless. But then you add in the fact
          that I had the audacity to have just
          graduated from an Ivy League
          school . . .

My finger pauses at a leather-bound book. I tip it over
the edge to the floor. THUNK.

                    ME
     . . . that I had innovative ideas for
     the curriculum . . .

Down goes another book. THUNK.

                    ME
     . . . that I had a charisma that they
     couldn't replicate . . .

THUNK.

                    ME
     . . . add all that up and I became a
     deadly threat to their comfortable
     little lives. "How dare he shine,"
     right?

I take a framed FACULTY PHOTO from the bookcase and walk
it slowly to Bill's desk.

                    ME
     So they chipped away at me every
     day. Forget learning from me or
     collaborating with me. They wanted me
     to shut up and dance. And I wouldn't
     do it. I kept fighting them. And every
     day they fought back harder. Stripping
     me away until I wasn't sure if I was
     even on the right side of this goddamn
     fight!

I SLAM the photo into the desk. Glass shards everywhere.
Bill anxiously looks to the door, hoping for an intrusion.
I play with the shards, calmly entranced.

> ME
>
> And that makes you feel crazy, Bill.
> Like your mind isn't your own. And
> when that happens, you might do what I
> did . . .

I grab a thin shard, make my way around the desk.

> ME
>
> . . . and learn what a panic
> attack is when you get picked up by
> an ambulance on I-90 because your body
> convinced you that you were going to
> die at the wheel.

I lean over, our faces inches apart. Sweat beads on
Bill's upper lip. I place a hand on the desk, just next
to his balled-up fist.

> ME
>
> So now I'm up to my eyeballs in
> prescription pills that make me feel
> even crazier. All so I can wake up
> every morning and be hated for trying
> to do a job I want so desperately to
> love.

I STAB the shard down into the flesh between my thumb and
forefinger. Blood blooms. Bill flinches and tries to look
away but I grab his face with my free hand. We're eye to
eye.

> ME
>
> I am quitting because this community
> hates me. And I think I'm starting to
> hate myself.

I pull the shard from my hand, regard it for a moment, then fling it onto the desk.

                    ME
          Is that enough for you to grow from,
          Bill?

CLOSE-UP on my eyes, sparked with madness, dulled by Xanax, gaze falling back to the floor in defeat as we JUMP BACK TO—

INT. ANOTHER HEADMASTER'S OFFICE—2006—DAY

                    BILL
          May I ask why you feel you need to
          leave?

My eyes lift slowly and we see that they are hollow, life-less. Desperate.

<u>No trace of the righteous madness of my glass shard-laden</u>
<u>daydream.</u>

                    ME
          (barely audible, almost catatonic)
          Tired. I'm tired of fighting. I was
          never the right fit here. And now I'm
          unfit to be anywhere.

                                              CUT TO:

INT. MED SCHOOL LECTURE HALL—2008—DAY

One hundred twenty future doctors mill about, finding their seats. Four Black faces in the lot, including ME (mid-20s, strong goatee) checking my phone in the back row.

RICH (mid-20s, Black face number five) sits down
next to me in a show of animated agitation. He glowers
in silence.

                         ME
             So I guess this is when I ask if you
             want to talk about it?

                         RICH
             Man, fuck that dude.

                         ME
             Sure. Whoever he is, fuck him.

                         RICH
             So I walk in the building five minutes
             ago and the dean sees me and pulls me
             aside. He's all, "Hey, Rich, great to
             see you, but hey, listen. Your hair.
             Very cool, but like I say, 'This ain't
             college.' It doesn't quite meet our
             standards of professionalism."

I take in Rich's modest blowout fade mohawk. It's fresh
as hell. In no way obscene. Rich rounds on me.

                         RICH
             He never came out and said it
             but . . . Is he even allowed to make
             me cut my hair?

                         ME
                       (shrugging)
             No idea.

                    RICH
Man, fuck this. And fuck him. I'm 'bout
to make so much noise about this shit.
I'm talking going over his head and
scaring the shit out of the powers
that be. I'm talking going online and
lighting this whole fucking school up.

                    ME
Those are . . . yeah, those are options.

                    RICH
Okay, okay, maybe don't scorch all of
the earth. But dude, we're being
targeted. They'd never ask fuckin'
White Boy Jared over there to trim his
goddamn surfer hair, you feel me?

Rich heaves a sigh and collapses deep into his seat.

                    RICH
    What do you think?

I take a look around the hall: the demographics, the
gleaming new desks, the marble trim, the state-of-the-
art interior design. A tottering, bespectacled PROFESSOR
steps to the podium. Students take their seats.

                    ME
                (to myself)
    Fuck. We're too far from home.

                    RICH
    What was that?

                    ME
    Just cut it, dude.

We lock eyes. Righteous indignation versus compromised survival. And in the end, disappointment. In ourselves. In each other.

The Professor taps the mic, calling the room to order.

Rich and I turn our attention forward. Nothing more to say.

                                                    CUT TO:

INT. DETROIT HOSPITAL OPERATING ROOM—EARLY 2010S—DAY

Bright lights. A draped body lies on a cold table. Neck exposed, filleted open. Three men, gowned and gloved, stand over the open wound: the diminutive DR. YAN, perched on a step stool, holds a suction tool as KENNY (senior resident) dissects carefully.

The last man, of course, is ME (hipster-adjacent glasses taped to my forehead). I sway a bit while holding a retractor. Dr. Yan clocks it.

                    DR. YAN
          Everything all right?

                    ME
          Actually, I really don't feel too
          great. Been feeling sick to my stomach
          all day.

Kenny And Dr. Yan share a momentary glance.

                    DR. YAN
          Oh boy. Well, we don't need you passing
          out or vomiting into the neck, so why
          don't you go take a break?

                              ME
          Yes, sir. Thanks.

I step away, rip off my gown, steady myself against waves
of nausea and step into—

**INT. DETROIT HOSPITAL O.R. HALLWAY—EARLY 2010S—
MOMENTS LATER**

I lower my mask and suck in a deep breath, let it out
slowly. I take one step and stop. LAUGHTER, MURMURS,
the MUFFLED SOUND OF MY NAME are heard through the OR
door.

I shake my head. That couldn't be. Mind playing tricks.

I stagger on to the restroom.

                                              CUT TO:

INT. DETROIT BANQUET HALL—EARLY 2010S—EVENING

LAUGHTER rolls through a sharply dressed crowd.
Chandeliers. Gilded sconces. Elegant place settings.
Full wineglasses.

IRA GOLDING (late 20s, junior resident, born for the
spotlight) stands behind a podium that bears a large
sign: OTOLARYNGOLOGY DEPT. GRADUATION DINNER.

                              IRA
          Oh yes, nobody is safe this evening.
          The roast must roll on, and the next
          victim is our very own Dr. Chin-Quee.

My smiling face fills the screen behind Ira's podium.

At the back of the hall we find ME (suit slightly too
small, dress shoes have seen better days) awaiting a
cocktail at the bar. I turn at the sound of my name.

                          IRA
          We all know he's a ladies' man. I've
          seen him at work. He's incredible. Now,
          I don't know about you, but I just
          can't believe that he's never sired a
          child in his life of wild
          transgressions.

Chuckles break out in the crowd. I take a long sip of my
drink, eyes on Ira.

                          IRA
          So I took the liberty of running his
          DNA through a database of all children
          born in the U.S. and surrounding
          territories since Tony turned 16.

A new slide fills the screen: a map of the U.S. dotted
with tiny pictures of MY FACE WITH BABY BOWS ON TOP in
each state. Twice in Florida.

The crowd—my bosses, coworkers, and colleagues—erupt in
MANIC LAUGHTER.

                          IRA
          I guess we know where his checks will
          be going after he graduates in a
          couple of years!

More laughter. Heads swivel, searching for me, hungry for
my reaction.

I sip my drink, smile broadly, raise my glass in a toast
to Ira.

                          IRA
          All right, moving on to our graduating
          seniors . . .

I down my drink in one swig, smile still plastered on my face. I nod at the BARTENDER; she refills my glass.

CUT TO:

INT. DETROIT HOSPITAL HALLWAY—EARLY 2010S—MORNING

A door swings closed. The affixed nameplate reads THE GENERAL—PROGRAM DIRECTOR. A hand pulls it shut with a CLICK.

It's ME. Once again. Soiled, baggy, sweat-stained scrubs. Head hung low, eyes drooping, fighting sleep as I contemplate my latest admonishment.

My head snaps up, staving off sleep. I move in an exhausted daze to the resident room door, nearly barreling into PEYTON.

PEYTON

Hey.

ME

Hey.

He opens the door and I follow into—

INT. DETROIT HOSPITAL RESIDENT ROOM—CONTINUOUS

A locker room with desks and computers. Bags and winter jackets line the scant wall space. Paperwork sits in sloppy piles all around.

Peyton takes a chair and starts typing away. I pull a peacoat from a hook and slip it on.

I tug on the zipper and it sticks. I try again. The zipper breaks.

ME
(to myself)

Fuck.

I regroup, try fastening the buttons. The top button comes loose, falls to the carpet.

                                    ME
                              (to myself)
                         God fucking damn it.

I look up to find Peyton silently observing this devastatingly minor struggle. Our eyes meet. He sees the exhaustion, the anger, the defeat. He sees my resignation.

Peyton turns back to his screen. Clicks at his keyboard.

I nod. I've always known that this was where my status as Peyton's "friend" would lead.

Silence.

I take my leave. The door closes behind me. CLICK.

                                        FADE TO FUCKING BLACK

Well, at least one thing about me hasn't changed since I was a kid: movies still find a way to articulate what I cannot. And through this one, I can see that I've spent a lifetime losing sight of the plot. I was never a passive bystander, watching the world's injustices pass me by. I was a child of war, born under attack, enduring blow after blow, victimized under a sophisticated, invisible, and enduring form of age-old genocide. I was the object of the bloodlust and taste for mass murder on which this nation was built.

Fuck this racism shit, man. Goddamn.

It makes soldiers out of each and every melanated one of us. And we're never given a choice, are we? We're all awakened to the fact that we live in a war zone at some point early in our lives. Until then, we believe life is fair, that everyone plays by the same rules. And then we see a lynching. Or a body dragged behind a speeding pickup truck. Or a fresh corpse beneath a police officer's smoking gun barrel.

Or the event is quieter, subtler, more confusing, and ultimately more maddening.

I *knew* I was the valedictorian of my elementary school. I'd seen the grades and class rankings just days before. There'd been no *doubt*. But when I rushed to my parents after the ceremony, desperate to hear them say that I wasn't fucking crazy for believing I was the best student, they hesitated. It was just a moment. A quick, shared, anxious glance between them as they weighed whether it was more harmful to plant seeds of doubt regarding my intelligence in my mind or tell me the truth that the game—hell, my entire life—had been rigged against me. Is there a right time to shatter the illusion of childhood's safe and limitless magic?

"It was almost you. Next time you just need to work harder. Leave no doubt."

They chose to lie. But their blinks of hesitation had already broken childhood.

I was awakened. In a war zone. Age ten.

As much as I know they wanted to shield me from the racist realities of the world, they ultimately failed. Primarily because they couldn't shield me from the internalized savage tendencies their own battles had left them. My father rarely shared the details of his life with me, and when he did, they were conspicuously abridged. For example, when I was in grade school he told me that he'd lived in Indiana for a year. That's where he'd started law school. But he'd finished his final two years of school in New York. And that was the whole story. No matter how many questions I asked, he made it clear that that year of his life was strictly off-limits to me.

Only after several years of overheard snippets of hushed conversations did I learn the truth.

My father thanked God often for his sprinter's thighs and strong lungs. Without them he wouldn't have escaped with his life on the many afternoons he'd spent fleeing on foot down residential streets, pursued by a speeding pickup truck with murderous intent. All for the crime of living on the wrong side of town.

He was also a light sleeper and woke one night not to shadows and moonlight but to a room bathed in an unnatural orange, its source flickering just outside his window: a cross crackling in flames on his front lawn. He'd wanted to yell for help but saw quickly that dispassionate eyes watched from every neighbor's window. He could expect no aid from those shadowed faces. They likely wanted to watch him burn as well.

Fueled by the secret truths of those midwestern days and nights, he taught me life lessons clouded by pain, laced with spite and anger. *I could be his revenge. I'd be no victim. I'd be the one who hunted. I'd be the predator who might one day rob his tormentors' daughters of innocence and agency. White girls were for practice. Because they needed to pay for the sins of their fathers.*

So I grew up—anger and defeat the undercurrents of the lessons I learned at home; constant reminders of the power I didn't have whenever I stepped out into the world. All I wished for was control. Over anything. As all teens do. I found a measure of it in my handful of Black friendships, those of us who made up the quota in my 97 percent white private school. We didn't always like one another, having been forced into camaraderie by skin color and not personality, but sometimes our shared experience was all we had. And the one thing we could control was the way we navigated the absurdities of discrimination. There was strength in that. Power. We didn't want to be saved by anyone. Never looked to be, no matter how many taxis refused to stop for us. We could laugh about it in the winter's cold because we weren't alone.

And somehow, even though we had nothing, we managed to get robbed one night. By a white lady who was trying her best to "do the right thing." Trying so hard that she looked right past the fact that in weaponizing her audacity and visibility and power against blatant racism *without our permission*, she only managed to infantilize us. I learned another isolating lesson that night about this war I'd been born into: I'd rather freeze than be saved by one of the "good ones."

That night made me bold. I wanted to fight and be heard. Maybe even be feared. So I set my sights on my school, full of good white people who only ever wanted to play nice and appear magnanimous, and fucking scorched the earth. I relished every stuttering response, every set of ashamed red cheeks, every pitiful tear. I drowned them in the uncomfortable repercussions of admitting me—a safe, diverse, token student—into their halls. Fuck the consequences. It felt incredible, intoxicating. It felt so great that I became recklessly confident enough to start lashing out at the asshole white people too.

Then they all fought back. And I was not ready.

At first it was overt. Verbal abuse and threats of violence. N-words and monkey slurs and lies to the police. All tactics I could accept and keep fighting. It was war, after all. They'd done the same to my family and friends for my entire life and we were all still standing.

But then the battleground changed. Whiteness penetrated my mind, where I was already fragile and defenseless. In my head, which was already full of fucked-up voices, whiteness never spoke but nudged my own thoughts in a direction that suited its goals: they'd made a mistake hiring me as an educator right out of college because I wasn't a good teacher; I wasn't a good teacher because I didn't follow the rules; if I didn't follow the rules, I didn't belong; I didn't belong, so I was alone; if I was alone, I couldn't succeed; if I couldn't succeed, I should just quit.

Whiteness stole my will to fight, choked my rebellious voice down to a whisper, made giving up seem like the only option and, seeing as it was a silent, invisible force in my mind, convinced me that it was all *my* choice. *My* idea. *My* weakness and inadequacy. Because like depression, racism's greatest trick is convincing you that it doesn't exist.

The white people in that school hated me so fucking much for entering their world. And they got their wish. They broke my fighting spirit.

I raised a white flag. Let me go or take me prisoner, I thought, just don't make me fight anymore.

Then I started medical school.

The most devastating consequence of giving up was the acceptance that my survival hinged on my internalization of the inevitability, the unstoppable force of white supremacy. I entered the world of medicine thinking not that I'd achieve all I was capable of but that I'd take as much success as white people would allow me. Their rules were law, and I'd follow them. I'd adopt any behavior that I knew would make them comfortable—emulate their handshakes and smiles and self-important laughter. I'd never give them cause for alarm. From me or any other Black face. I'd encourage all of us to give up. It was the only way we could ensure our safety. The only way to eke out any measure of hollow success, whatever that meant.

I did all of those things. And still, despite my surrender, white people hunted me.

They took knives to my already faltering confidence with suggestions that I adjust my professional expectations, set my sights on specialties that I could "realistically handle." Insinuated that I must be too lazy to study any time I offered an incorrect answer on the wards. Skewered my reputation by laughing behind closed doors about how I must be showing up to work hungover when I was ill. Carved away at my sanity by convincing me that Peyton simply *knew instinctively* how to do the job better than I did. He always knew the expectations. Always happened to be right where he needed to be. Always seemed to have banked enough goodwill to have his mistakes forgiven with a shrug or an encouraging pat on the back. There *had* to be some secret handbook he studied.

Some mentor whispering in his ear. But the bosses assured me that Peyton didn't need a helping hand to figure out the basics—he just *got it*. And Peyton himself? He never refuted these claims in my presence. He always seemed to prefer silence around me. Cool friendship, bro.

I'd left the battlefield and still they found ways to poke and prod and stab and slice until I was bled dry of any power I might have left in my veins. Without my knowing it, I began to reach out vindictively for control in any way I could. And the easiest way to do that was by sleeping with women. White women, to be specific. Almost exclusively. Because fuck their feelings. Every bead of sweat and fingernail scratch gouged into my back and scream of my name tasted of power. And revenge. One bold blonde even let pleasure push her so thoughtlessly far that she called me "nigger" as she rode on top of me. And though my mind immediately rang with rage and warnings, all was overridden by how much . . . I *loved* it. In the days that followed, I juggled self-disgust and self-satisfaction in equal confusing measure as I tried to make sense of my reaction. Then all became clear when a ballroom full of surgeons at a professional function laughed their asses off at the idea that I'd been fathering illegitimate children across the country since I was sixteen.

I laughed right along with them. Because despite every facet of my life that they'd lorded over for decades, every shred of innocence and safety and dignity that they'd robbed me of, I was fucking their daughters. And sisters. And mothers. And ex-wives and girlfriends. And those ladies couldn't get enough of the monkey whose humanity they toyed with for their amusement.

I'd become the revenge tool my father had always wanted. And the animal white people had always thought me to be.

And so I was for years. Powerless and misogynist and bleeding. And starving. For what I'd long since told myself was out of my reach.

Until this morning, when I nearly broke Dr. Krohn's jaw, blinded him in his own blood, and crushed his windpipe under my worn, peeling Danskos. Something new surged through me upon experiencing how confidently and loudly and publicly he thought he could treat me like a pet dog. My silence and submission had allowed this, had allowed these white folks to grow so bold as to throw off their masks of civility and show their true colors to the world without fear.

Fuck that shit. Not anymore.

Fuck yes. I've got to tell you, I've wondered for your entire life what real anger would look like on you. I'm into it.

Well, it's all very new, but I learned down in Mexico that anger, when released, won't consume me, as I always thought. It might be time to harness it and do something—

Constructive? Aggressive? Loud? Wild and unexpected?

I was thinking . . . *equal.* My spirit is finally ready to fight again. But this time, I'm fighting exactly as white people have shown me to: mercilessly, systematically, intelligently, and dirty as fuck.

A crisp autumn breeze whistled through the parking structure, filling my car with the refreshing scent of September in Detroit. Reclined in the driver's seat, eyes on the swift, low-hanging cloud cover, I exhaled slowly, reached for the keys, and turned off the engine. I was two hours removed from my standoff with Dr. Krohn, and surprisingly, I found my mind at peace. Peace and . . . something else. Was it comfort? Control? Clarity? Whatever the combination of emotions was, it brought the day's adventure into curious perspective.

A life's worth of moments—outright aggression, passive slights, inherited trauma, psychological torment—wrapped their tentacles around an idea I'd initially deemed silly and squeezed, churning opinion into hard fact: the institution of academic medicine was a stunningly faithful microcosm of the story of American white supremacy.

I smiled and sent my seat back into a slow recline as I let revisionist history wash over me.

It's no secret that the American medical profession is the province of the learned white man, founded on the premise of the white man's burden: due to his superior intellect, it was his duty to wield his knowledge for the greater good of society. All the world—all people of all colors, cultures, and creeds—was his domain. His patients were his loyal, downtrodden subjects. He'd calmly and rationally persuade them to sacrifice their minds and bodies at his altar, all in the name of innovation, experimentation, science, and the health and betterment of the many. They'd oblige without question—he was so smart, so self-assured, so *noble*. They'd offer him their blood and revere him for the opportunity. They loved him. And oh, how he loved himself.

Eventually the tides of society shifted, and those he'd claimed dominion over came knocking at his door—not to be saved but to learn so that they might share in his bounty. Women. All manner of melanin-infused faces. The inferior sex and the help. Preposterous. It was he who had singularly and meticulously garnered the power to save lives. Why would he share it?

But he'd taken a Hippocratic oath of beneficence, of generosity. He had to do *something*—the eyes of the world were upon him. So he allowed us, the *others*, incremental steps forward and disguised them as mighty gifts. We were admitted to his hallowed halls but were neglected once we arrived. He held us to unfamiliar rituals of decorum and narrow, strangely specific standards of excellence that most of our fair-skinned, male colleagues seemed to know and understand instinctively. In essence, we were expected (but never asked—he'd never say it out loud) to do our best white-boy impression in order to survive. And even if some of us figured out *what* he wanted us to be, he never overtly shared the secrets of *how* to achieve the coveted white-boy status.

So the outside world rejoiced at the noble progress made within our profession. We, the others, marveled at the achievement of simply existing within the walls of the profession. And all the while the White Man Doctor knew that the true keys to the castle, the password to the secret society of learned men who made the real decisions and truly guided the profession, were locked securely away from us. He'd never speak the truth out loud—that no matter how hard we tried to act like him, he would never allow us to *be* him.

The discrimination was invisible, impossible to prove, and so could never be fought. His power was secure for generations to come.

It was brilliant.

So to the learned white man I say, respectfully, well done.

Now, feel free to fuck off.

Because I see you. Your secrets are no longer safe.

For my entire life I've been forced to study whiteness. I didn't want to, and never asked to be enrolled in the curriculum, but I didn't have a choice—in this world my aspirations, my limitations, my health and safety all depended on it. Every interaction with white people, benign or malignant, has been academic. Good thing I'm a good-ass student. So good, in fact, that I found the fatal flaw in the veneer of whiteness and, thanks to my recent dose of the *Tonydon'tgiveafuckaboutyofeelingscuzhefinallylookingout forhisownyoutrickbitch* vaccine, I plan on targeting that weakness and kicking the shit out of it.

In my estimation, the Achilles' heel of whiteness is that, for all of its power and control, it is as fragile as an eggshell. And this fragility stems from the fact that whiteness is the cornerstone of white folks' self-image. Unfortunately for them, that cornerstone's strength is predicated upon the belief that they are right to hold whatever power and privilege they possess, and that they are innocent of any wrongdoing that might have made that status possible.

They must be *right* and they must be *innocent*.

If somehow the idea that either of these two things is in doubt seeps into their minds, their eyes go wide, blood rushes from their nose- and earholes, and they tearfully admit that the friends from *Friends* weren't actually very good friends to one another at all. And then their heads explode.

Or, like, the existential crisis equivalent.

Where it gets tricky is in the fact that white people often subconsciously know just how fragile their self-image actually is. So when they feel the truth of their relationship to whiteness come under attack, their defense mechanisms mount in force. This is when indignation sparks, leading to anger and resolving in violence. This is when white tears fall in rivers, making victims of aggressors and oppressors. This is when they tell you about their Black husband, wife, or friend. This is when they pass laws and uphold social conventions to gaslight you into believing that the world is fair, and that you just need to work harder to achieve what they were given. This is when they take a knee or raise a fist to protest in public solidarity in the name of your life's worth, but then can't seem to find the time in their schedules to sit down and build the system that would protect you from harm.

Very, very tricky.

But a new war tactic spun in the air, nestled between the sweet perfume of autumn leaves and the stagnant fumes of car exhaust, as I lay reclined in my little Japanese sedan. Whiteness—white power, white supremacy, white saviorism, white burdens, white privilege, white innocence—had always been immune to full frontal attack. But as I'd learned in my own experience, war is never fully waged in the field before our eyes. The most brutal and effective attacks are those that are hurled and detonated in the dark, quiet recesses of our minds. The ones that shake our deepest foundations, leaving us to question who we are and what we are truly fighting for.

What if I could wage a covert operation to detonate oppressive whiteness? Plant seeds of doubt and confusion so subtly and skillfully that white people think that *they planted those seeds themselves*?

Now *that's* an idea.

I could lead them into conversations, cultural celebrations, public protests, family gatherings, and even patient interactions—any situation in which their perspective isn't centered as the default. White people really hate that shit. Then I could contrive to keep them there *just* a bit longer than they think they can handle. And when they inevitably squirm under the uncomfortable truths of the fucked-up cascading consequences of their innocence, blind spots, and uninterrogated beliefs and choices, they'll look to me. They'll hope that I'll be the cog in their defense mechanism that

I've always been and absolve them of the intrusive feelings of guilt, shame, and wrongdoing.

Unfortunately, I won't be playing that shit anymore. I'll smile politely and calmly say some variation of "No, bitch. The best thing I can do for you is leave you to bathe in those feelings, and allow your fragile little mind to spin until your life's worth of rationalizations turn to dust."

And then I'll do it again. I'll do it until they decide that they want to, *need to*, do something about their perspective in order to look themselves in the mirror. Because white people won't do shit, know they *don't have to do shit*, unless they *want* to.

And I'll teach this new art of war to all of my partners-in-arms—the unseen, silenced, trod upon, and forgotten. Together we will awaken to the life-affirming certainty that, despite what they've made us believe, we are not alone. And that the strength to fight for our humanity lies even deeper than our bones. Each of us will devise our own unique tactics, find myriad ways to invade their minds. All the better to catch them increasingly off guard.

And then we will strike again. And again. And again.

And one day, the dam will break. Whiteness will find its face splintered. And white people will only know and understand that they did it to themselves.

And their fragile self-imagery will collapse in one of two ways.

First, the would-be allies. The Peytons of the world who want to believe themselves to be good and kind and generous but spent a lifetime handcuffed by their own cowardice. They'll find themselves in search of atonement, of education in how to right the wrongs they've wrought, and of a friendly hand to hold along the way. Their search will lead them to me: the kind one with the big smile and an appreciation of the Beatles and *Seinfeld* who'd always made them feel (almost) comfortable. They'll confess that they'd stood in the rooms I wasn't invited into. That they sat idly by as I was doubted, denigrated, and laughed at in these white spaces. That they rationalized their silence to me by telling themselves that they were protecting me, shielding me from the toxicity. That they wished they'd had the courage to stand up when it counted, but they were here now and could no longer live with themselves if they couldn't make it right. They'll hope desperately for my forgiveness.

And I will refuse to give it to them.

As for an education on how to do better? I'll tell them to go read a goddamn book. Because I am not their teacher. Just as I had to learn the truth on my own, they can do the same. And even though they previously left me to feel as if I were losing my mind, hearing whispers and voices that I couldn't prove existed, I won't do the same. I'll validate their feelings, the reality of their experience. And I'll happily answer their questions once they've done the fucking work.

Because *that's* what a real friend does, Peyton.

And what of the ultimate question? What's the answer when white people have done the research and the soul-searching and their "good person" egos hang by a thread and they wonder what they can do to help us emerge from the centuries of brutality they've created and benefited from? I'm sure plenty of brilliant thinkers smarter than me have explored this for ages. But in my mind, it's pretty simple. The easy answer we tend to give is "Hey, <insert white name here>, you should focus on using your power and privilege to help lift up those less fortunate." But that's wrong. It still puts white people at the center of the universe and sends us right back to square one.

What I plan to say is "Hey, *<insert even whiter name here>*, now that you finally recognize the power you have, impress me and earn my trust by giving it up. We don't want you to bestow anything on us. We want a trade: you lift us higher by bringing yourself lower. Make yourself humble. Make yourself poorer. Make yourself weaker. Make yourself vulnerable. All in the name of equally sharing this world with someone who doesn't look, speak, or act like you for once in your fucking life. That would be a start."

I have a feeling that the good white people, the real allies, will do exactly as I say. They'll give up their power freely. They'll want to. Because it will seem the only way to uphold their fragile self-image.

And then there are the proud. The stubborn. The Dr. Krohns. The ones who want what they believe they've earned and achieved but, in the face of my cheerfully brutal war tactics, will suddenly find themselves stymied by the moral ambiguity of the means. Their faith in themselves will stand on a newly shaky foundation, but they'll never willingly give up their power.

And I won't ask them.

Because the time will have come to just take that shit myself.

By force.

Emboldened by my Black-ass manifesto, I returned my car seat back to its upright and locked position, pulled my phone from a scrub chest pocket, and dialed.

"Yes?" Dr. Krohn puffed into the receiver.

"Hey, Dr. Krohn, it's Tony. I just wanted to follow up with you about this morning."

No response. Only the comically loud big-bad-wolf breaths he regularly used to intimidate. *This fucking guy.*

"Right, well, I wanted to apologize if I unintentionally offended this morning. I was doing my best to take ownership of our patient and act in his best medical, personal, and financial interests. You've told me on several occasions that these are the expectations of a senior resident."

Huff, Puff.

"My point, sir, is that I'm here to learn from you. But as I progress through training, the nature of our educational interactions will change. I will question and challenge you more in order to make myself better, just as I expect you will do for me. I just hope that we can continue to foster an environment where it's safe for trainees to ask questions and take risks in order to grow."

Silence.

"Anyway, I hope you have a great day. I'll see you tomorrow morning for rounds."

Nothing. Oh well. I moved to end the call when—

"Yes," murmured Dr. Krohn in a faraway whisper, "I'll see you tomorrow."

And so I tipped over the first domino.

At some point Dr. Krohn's anger would give way to the shame of a trainee twenty years his junior taking it upon himself to be the bigger man and pick up the phone. He'd wish that he could have bristled at and dismissed his student's petulance, but instead he'd find himself set off-balance by the resident's calm clarity. Though he couldn't yet explain it, something in his world was no longer quite right.

That is exactly where I wanted him.

And when the time ultimately came to usurp his power, I'd be ready to take it through whatever degree of violence I saw fit.

Motherfucker.

I sped home, knowing that I'd just lit the match that would ignite a new phase in the war for my humanity—this time on a battlefield of my own making. The freedom to be defined not by my endurance to suffering but by *literally anything else* coursed through my veins.

Black was so much more than pain.

And if I had my way, the world would see it, marvel at it, revere it, and protect it.

Goddamn. Lofty goals.

As soon as I walked into my sad little apartment, I found myself moved to gather dozens of pages of loose scrap paper, a pen, and a set of headphones. I pressed play on a triumphant Lil Wayne instrumental—soaring strings and bouncing horns and snapping snares and 808s—and let my pen take me away. Rhythmic bars in the vein of my street-corner Brooklyn ancestors spilled out with an urgency that caught me by surprise. I had never been one for songwriting, but after the revelations of the day, I felt I no longer had a choice.

This latest leg in my journey will be long and arduous. It might even last the rest of my life. I'll undoubtedly find myself in quiet moments of doubt. But never on my knees in surrender.

Never again.

My heart's rhythm of righteousness and resilience and uncaged power will march on, inviting the spirits of all for whom and with whom I fight to sing their melodies.

I can hear them even now.

Even as my pen runs dry.

Friends and strangers.

Even as I press a pencil to the nub.

Family. Father. And ancestors.

Even if I have to punctuate the last verse with my own blood.

I can't stop.

I won't stop.

Because every revolution needs its rebel music:

Y'aint no
Valedictorian by default,
    all because Jason Finklestein took the last day off.
Y'aint know
That the chick you into just got two dates,
    until her parents try to break her out this "hood phase."
Y'aint know
That little Katie who kissed you in kindergarten
Would get all grown up, on a Sunday night she was joggin'
Through gentrified Brooklyn where quarter waters have
    become lattes.
She turns the corner and she sees you, you can read
    her face.
Cross the street? Nah—too much traffic, it's not clear.
About face? But her mama told her we smell fear.
So she rummages in her pocketbook,
    palms are sweating she drops
    both her mace and car keys her time is up
    and she sees
She can't go.
Her feet are frozen, praying that God guards her, and you?
Y'aint no Pooh Bear but you ain't no monster
As you hand her back what she would use to blind you when
    you come near.
    Hm.
        Maybe she deserves that fear.

Y'aint know
That they need a token, currency that shows them how to
        shine
And it's you. Tony remember all you do with pride
Is being packaged for masters, helping them sleep
        at night
Until they wake from their slumber because their
        windpipe
Is being crushed by the monkey that they let inside
The big house. Thought all I did was dance? Nah, sike.
They let a beast out the cage,
        and taught him that he craves a stage
        so that mothers, brothers, and sisters
            will all learn how to fly.

Cuz ain't no man tannin', no sleepin' and eatin'
When you command respect it's also their resentment you're
        feeding
I live today like it's the eve of my own assassination
        You can't know.
        You ain't no—
I said it ain't no man tannin', no sleepin' and eatin'
When you command respect it's also their resentment you're
        feeding
I live today like it's the eve of my own assassination
        You can't know (so set them ablaze).
        You ain't no (no, no no) . . .

Y'aint no
        slave
                to the sins of your father.
His blood is in your veins,
        his weakness it haunts ya.

His demons whisper you lullabies more and more
And now their voices are starting to sound a lot like yours:

"Manipulate your kids,
And blind them so they never start to get to questioning,
Or breaking down all of your flaws. Ignore the warning
    signs,
Go head get married under pressure
Then you leave her,
    find a new one,
    leave your offspring to fend for
Themselves but not before you teach them that white girls are
    for practice,
Discount their feelings, their intelligence, doubt their
    intentions,
To get your subtle revenge
        on those pickup truck–driving rednecks
                who lit your lawn on fire
                        just for being Black in the Midwest."

    Lord.

Took thirty years, but I understand
    the fear of raising a man, when you're a broken man.
Am I wrong for wanting to find my baby a white mama?
Alienate him from my pain and hope his light-skinned life is
    calmer?
Would my mama cry when she heard the things that
    I ponder?
And think I never found the beauty in her hair, and
    skin color?
Or could she see what I see:
This world was never meant for me

How do I leave my legacy if I get shot down in these streets
toni—[*pop pop pop* of deadly gunshots]

Y'aint know
Fear is setting in because you finally found your wings
They always said the sky is blue beyond that transparent
    ceiling
And you believed them until now, cuz this glass room is not
    for you
Take a sledgehammer to that roof and find the sky's not even
    blue
The heavens open up for you,
    beyond the atmospheric hue,
You kiss the sun, the stars, the moon,
    the earth is fading out of view
Your lungs fill deeper than you knew
    they had the capacity to
        and then you finally know the truth.

Y'aint no child martyr.
Count my breaths, not my blessings. These streets are wild,
    Mama.
Do I matter when my killer escapes his trial, Mama?
Fingers wrapping around my neck and not your smile, Mama,
    are the last things I ever see.

Y'aint no role model.
Glocks in 'raris, hotline blinging, whip and nae nae, and rich
    homies making women
    drink out of gold bottles.
Hijack the visions of dreamers,
    adolescent believers
Don't tell them when you sell your mind and body, your soul
    follows.

Y'aint no dreamin' southern reverend who ain't know better,
    marched on the capital but brought the clap home to
        Coretta.
Y'aint no Detroit Red whose disciples' Beretta vendetta split
    his head—
    the only way he'd be remembered forever.

Y'ain't know that I raised your babies when you weren't able
    you is kind, you is smart, but took my dinner in the stable.
Y'ain't no light-skin fiddler finna wait till Massuh sleeps
    Bring your family his muskets and cutlery
        cuz the revolution finna start with ME!

No arms. No legs.
    they atrophy when you're packed side to side, head to feet
        and
No God. No faith.
    forsaken by all that you once believed cuz
No light. All day.
    as you rise and fall on a never-ending sea
You smell decay of the body of your brother next to you, he's
    been dead two weeks
But
That's not your fate.
    cuz the blood in your veins is the blood of a king.
You'll live today and tomorrow and forever in the eyes of all
    your offspring,
Tell 'em
Chain me, and whip me, and rape me but you'll never see
    me cry.
Make laws to equally separate me,
    then watch me rise.
And
When it's 1983 and a baby's born and he looks like me

and he don't know his history
        cuz he lacks a father figure
Tell him, "You are legacy.
        progeny of royalty.
                they will fear you when you sleep
                        cuz you always dream bigger
You will transcend the prison of minds in defeat
And you'll finally be free because
        you
        ain't
        no

                                nigga."

EIGHT

FATHERHOOD

JAZLYN

"FAAAAAAAACK!"

I reclined in my chair, squeezing my eyes shut with my hands, once again amazed by the instant relief a well-prolonged expletive can give. Weight shifted in the chair to my right as it spun toward me.

"Hoo boy," said Jazlyn, "that was a nice long one. What happened this time?"

I uncovered my eyes and spun my chair wearily to face her. Jazlyn was two years my junior and always looked at me with the playful eagerness of one who desperately wanted to be in on the next joke, whatever it might be. It was totally endearing. And it drove me completely insane.

"Did you receive the latest angry-gram about you from the boss?" I asked.

Her eyebrows shot up. "What! I haven't even yelled at anybody for the last two weeks!"

I let out a long sigh. "Do you want a dramatic reading?"

"Ugh. Sure," she said as she leaned back and set herself spinning. I scooted back to my computer screen. It was Friday afternoon, and the resident workroom was deserted but for the two of us.

"'Dear General, I am writing to inform you that I've received another complaint about an interaction with one of your residents: Jazlyn Bacani—'"

"Hey, that's me!"

"Missing the point. Pay attention, please." I returned my gaze to the screen. "'One of my nurses reported that she paged Dr. Bacani last week to let her know that she'd been unable to place an IV access in a patient.'"

Jazlyn chuckled dismissively to herself and turned back to her snack.

"'Dr. Bacani then asked her where she'd gone to nursing school, and followed up by asking if the school was real or if she'd taken classes online.' Holy shit, dude. I'm not condoning it, but that's an objectively sick burn."

Jazlyn shrugged and continued munching on a mouthful of granola.

I went on. "'She then continued to berate my nurse, calling into question her skills and knowledge base. Ultimately, Dr. Bacani came to see the patient and placed the IV access, all while telling my nurse that she should never have to call a doctor to place an IV. I only learned of this interaction when I found this nurse in the break room, distraught and crying.'"

"Oh, get the fuck out of here," Jazlyn garbled through a mouth filled with half-chewed walnuts. I motioned for her to swallow, for the sake of intelligibility and relative classiness. She gulped hard and continued. "Crying? In the break room? The only reason anyone ever cries in the break room is to get attention. Cry silently on the toilet like a fucking grown-up."

I pushed on. "'I kindly ask that you address this behavior with Dr. Bacani, as she has, on more than one occasion, had adversarial interactions with our staff and contributed to an environment that several nurses feel is hostile. Sincerely, Arlene McDonald, nursing supervisor.'"

I swung my chair around and studied her. Though she was two years behind me in training, we were actually the same age. We were both atypically old for our years, as we'd both lived atypically interesting lives in the years between college and medical school. As elder statespeople, the culture of the hospital and residency struck us as uniquely absurd. Our younger counterparts lacked perspective—we'd lived and worked in the real world before this journey. Life in this hospital was not the real world. Life in this hospital was fucking ridiculous. Sadly, our broad perspective was not liberating—knowing the extent to which we were being broken down, beat up, and exploited took a particularly harsh toll on us. And in spite of Jazlyn's generally cheerful disposition, the cracks in the mask were starting to show.

I knew all about masks.

I raised my eyebrows, inviting any response to these charges of malicious emotional abuse in the workplace.

"I didn't even yell at her!" she cried.

"I know."

"And I'm not wrong!" She pulled her hair back and began tying it into a tight bun with the elastic band that she always kept on her wrist—one of her telltale signs of gearing up for a fight. "I used to be a floor nurse, and I know when a nurse is being fucking lazy!

You get the fucking IV placed. If it's hard, you ask other nurses with more experience to help you and you learn how they do it. You don't call the fucking doctor to bail you out when all you've done is try twice in each antecubital. That's not fucking nursing. It's fucking lazy. And fucking incompetent. FUCK, I'M STILL HUNGRY!"

In a fit of rage she balled up her now-empty Ziploc bag and threw it across the room to the trash. Nothing but net.

"Hey, Kobe, you're not wrong," I said.

"Who's Kobe?"

"Oh my God, I don't have the bandwidth right now to educate you on the troubling holes in your pop culture knowledge. You know damn well you could have communicated your frustration more effectively. People don't magically do better when you call them stupid. They do better when you show them how to do better. Preferably in person. And preferably not after you've already made them cry."

"Yeah, yeah, I know you're right," she conceded, slumping into her chair with a sudden look of exhaustion.

"Listen," I said, pulling my chair closer to her. "I'll talk to Arlene, smooth this over, let her know what we expect of nurses prior to calling us for situations like this. But you've got to start making a point of being nicer to people. Because they all talk, and you're already on thin ice, bro."

She sat straight up at that. "What do you mean? Like, with our department?"

"Yeah."

I read her mounting WTF response and cut her off before she could rage. "Okay. Real talk sesh. Right now. Because you're an adult, and you deserve to be treated like one. All of the issues with junior residents come from the bosses straight to me, and I've always thought they were bullshit, so I'd just try to guide you in the direction they wanted instead of telling you the specifics. I just didn't want you to get into your own head about it too much."

"What sort of stuff have they been saying?"

"Some of it is the normal griping about second-years: needs to read more, needs to think more broadly about her diagnoses, blah blah blah. The usual stuff everyone needs to improve on. But the bigger stuff centers around them thinking you're . . . difficult."

"How am I fucking difficult?" she said, shaking her head in honest disbelief.

"They think you're too loud. You smile at people even if you're having a day when you answer all of the questions wrong, so they don't think you're taking your job seriously. You don't know when to hold your tongue. You're not appropriately deferential."

She was still as a statue, eyes boring into me.

"They have a problem with your *personality*. Funny thing is, both you and Liam are the same year and have the same struggles with the medicine. But they're fine with his mood swings on bad days. Do you know the difference between the two of you?"

Her cheeks flushed. She knew the answer before I opened my mouth.

"Yeah, exactly," I said, leaning in. "You're not white. And you're a woman. A Filipino woman, who these fuckers think at first glance should be a nurse and not a doctor. None of this shit was built for you."

I watched her eyes come in and out of focus for a few moments as she flicked through countless experiences of the past two years through a newly focused lens. Then she threw her head back and erupted in a single haughty cackle.

"So . . . so, then . . ." she stammered, shaking her head. "Then what can I—"

Just then, her pager chirped and she snapped back to the reality of life in the hospital: work comes first. Figure yourself out on your own time. She hopped to the phone and I slid back to my desk, eavesdropping as I checked emails.

"Hi, this is ENT returning a page . . . Uh-huh . . . uh-huh . . . mm . . . And the patient is stable right now? Okay. So when you try to pop it in, there should be some resistance. Sometimes you've got to put your back into it and . . . Well, lube it up, then! I'm sure this isn't the first time you've heard that—"

She was rudely interrupted by the sound of my head slamming against the desk. Fucking kids these days and their dick jokes.

"What?" she mouthed.

"Just tell them you're coming down," I mouthed back. She rolled her eyes and followed directions.

I pulled my white coat from its wall hook as she hung up the phone. "Okay, go get the tackle box. I'm coming with you."

"Coming on a call with a junior? I'm honored."

"You're goddamn right you are. Now hurry up."

The elevator door opened and we stepped inside.

"Okay, let me flesh this out for you," I said as the doors closed. "There's an archetype that all of the bosses want you to embody. They never tell you what it is, but they punish you for not achieving it. And the punishments are all behind your back—they talk shit to each other, or to your senior residents, but never straight to your face. Then one day the General pulls you in and says, 'Hey, uh <*sniff*>, so you are dangerously close to being on <*sniff*> probation.' And then you're like, '<*sniff*> <*sniff*> Weird, smells like some fucked-up-ass bullshit in your office, old man.'"

"Awesome," Jazlyn sighed, uncharacteristically subdued as she watched the blinking lights that marked our descent. "So they're setting me up to fail."

I smiled at that. I'd been saying the same words of defeat to myself not long ago. "Actually, think of it more as they're not actively helping you succeed." I took the tackle box from her. She had a way of naturally holding it like a strapped handbag, the handle perched on her forearm near the crook of her elbow so that she could gesture with her hand. She started to protest as I grabbed it, but I waved her off. "This isn't chivalry. You're gonna give yourself tendonitis if you keep holding it like that."

The elevator dinged for the ground floor and we walked through the familiar labyrinth of humid linoleum hallways.

"They're not going to go out of their way to support you, and they won't give you the benefit of the doubt, because your name isn't White Dude O'Connell," I continued as our clogs echoed throughout the corridor. "Think about it: Doesn't it seem like Liam always kind of knows what he's supposed to be doing? Like he knows what the bosses want of him?"

"So you think they tell him what to do?" she asked, opening a set of doors with her key card.

"That's a definite possibility, but I'm not in that club, so who knows? All I know for sure is that they don't tell *you*."

We turned another corner and swung open another door.

"So they're setting me up to fail," she said again.

"Yes. But you're not going to."

I locked eyes with her before we pushed through the next set of double doors. "Because I failed first. And with what little power I've got, I'm not going to let it happen to you."

She furrowed her brow, pushed through the door, and walked on ahead of me, massaging her forearm. I followed, allowing her the space to absorb the realities of the hidden curriculum—the unwritten secrets to residency success that had been kept from us, and simultaneously used against us.

She stopped at the ER entrance. "So what do I do, boss?"

I motioned for her to take a seat with me on a nearby bench.

"Welp," I began, loosening my clogs so that they hung from my toes, "you've got to give them what they want. I learned the hard way that, more than anything, you've got to give them the personality that they're looking for."

She crossed her arms and legs, letting a clog dangle from her big toe. "But that's such bullshit."

"It sure is. You've got to create a work persona, and it may be the complete opposite of your real-life persona. Work Jazlyn keeps her mouth shut so that she doesn't let the insults slip out, no matter how much truth they are laced with. She doesn't ask personal questions of the bosses and only talks business. She smiles and laughs a lot less. She doesn't share stories of what she did over the weekend or last night at home unless they start with 'So, I was studying last night . . .'"

She appeared exhausted at the prospect. You and me both, kid.

"How to be better prepared for each of those fuckers in the OR and in clinic? I can teach you that. I've spent enough time with them to know their soft spots and pet peeves. But the main thing is that you have to be way less you and a little more cyborg. It's not fucking fair. And when we're grown-ups maybe we can change this shit. But for now, we control what's ours to control so that we can survive this shit. And that means playing the game they built."

We sat in still silence at that, watching the flurry of traffic in and out of the emergency room.

"That sounds pretty shitty," she muttered.

"You are correct," I replied.

"So if I'm toning down the Jazzy," she continued, placing her clog back on her heel, "and I'm here twenty hours a day, how do I not lose the real Jazlyn altogether?"

I smiled. It was like hearing my inner monologue spoken out loud for the first time.

"That, my friend, is what's *actually* most important. You've got to find the little ways in which you can boost yourself. You can't count on anyone else to do it for you—it'll be a really long time before any of the bosses tell you that you're doing a good job, even if you are. So you've got to find ways to remind yourself not only that you deserve to be here, but that it's really important that you *are* here—that your presence actually makes a difference. You can find those moments with your patients, of course. But I find that I hold on even tighter to the moments I find with people I used to barely even spare a glance to because I was so sad about my own shit."

"Ooh, ooh! Like the Black Guy Head Nod!" she exclaimed, bouncing on the bench.

"The fuck? Whatchu know 'bout the Black Guy Head Nod? Who's been educating you?"

"Oh my God, you do it all the time! Like, you'll be walking and literally *any* Black dude will walk past you, and nobody smiles but you both do this little nod like, *Hey, brotha, what's the haps?* Then you just keep walking and that's it!"

"Okay, I'm going to forgive that problematic impression because you noticed something that these white folks never see even though it's happening all around them. Just don't let that shit happen again."

"No problem, brotha!" she chimed, holding up her hand for a high five. "OMG, I'm KIDDING!"

"Just for that, I'm leaving your ass hanging," I said, standing up and grabbing the tackle box. She continued to hold up her hand in expectation, then replaced her toothy grin with an exaggerated scowl and lifted her chin in a subtle nod. Goddamn it. She'd studied the Black folks well. I hit her with a crisp high five out of grudging respect.

"But you get it though, right?" I went on as she smoothed her coat. "You've made it. You are a part of the most respected profession in the world. And even though the ones who hold the keys to the kingdom try to convince you that you're nothing special, your *people* fucking know how special you are without having to say a word. They're proud of you whether you know them or not."

"I got you," she said, pulling out her key card again to enter the ER. "I think this could be fun."

"Just don't appropriate our shit. There are plenty of Filipinos around. You can figure out your own thing."

"You know that Filipinos are the Black folks of East Asia, right?"

"We'll discuss false equivalencies at a later date."

We were greeted by the familiar smell of the ER as we pushed through the double doors—stagnantly stale but recently disinfected—and turned a couple of corners to reach the patient's stall. Jazz reached for the curtain, then hesitated.

"Shit, I almost forgot," she whispered. "Deferential. Would you like to lead the way to the patient's bed, my good sir?"

"Don't be an asshole," I whispered back. The constant din of the ER had a way of covering up the less family-friendly conversations, as long as they were kept to a dull roar.

"Hey, how about this?" I went on. "How about we *Chapski*[1] this together?"

"Yes, sir," she whispered back with a smile. She yanked the curtain open and boisterously introduced herself. "Hi, everybody, I'm Dr. Bacani with ENT. This is my assistant, Dr. Chin-Quee. He'll be in the corner."

Son of a bitch, she sure didn't waste time when it came to role-playing. I smiled at the ER resident and nurse and surveyed the situation quickly. The patient had a tracheostomy—a hole in the front of the neck leading directly to her windpipe. Most patients with a tracheostomy have a short, curved hard plastic tube that sits in the hole, keeping it open. When the tube is not there, the body will start to heal the hole over time, causing it to shrink until it disappears. This old lady had developed an infection that made her lungs weak, so she was sedated and on a breathing machine that was hooked up to her trach tube. Problem was, each time the ventilator heaved breath into her airway, half of the air would hiss out around the edges of her trach tube. She was stable now, sure, but she wouldn't last the night like this. She needed a larger tube.

I opened the tackle box and rummaged around to ready

1. Parenthetical aside for context: The verb *to Chapski* is defined as the act of having a junior doctor demonstrate more competence than their superior. The term originated years ago among the ENT residents as a snarky response to the presence of our sweaty, earlobe-hair-combing attending Dr. Chapman, whose lack of clinical skills was recognized by even the most junior trainees. He scared the shit out of us.

everything that I knew she'd need while keeping an ear out for Jazzy, who was already taking charge.

"All right, I see we've got her oxygen sats up to a hundred percent, so in a second we're going to hold the vent, disconnect, remove this trach tube, and place the larger one." She paused to check the name tag of the young nurse standing at the foot of the bed. "Ambrosio?"

The nurse nodded, already pulling on a pair of gloves.

"I'm going to need you to lube up the new trach tube and hand it to me as soon as I ask for it, and you," she continued, now addressing the distressed ER resident across from her, "you're in charge of the vent."

"Okay, uhhhh . . ." the resident muttered, turning to the ventilator's screen. Jazzy and I shared a quick look—this resident didn't know what the fuck she was doing. I could see a snarky comment forming on Jazzy's lips, and I pleaded with my eyes for her to take the high road.

"Are you a f— Are you, um, uncomfortable with that?" she spat out through gritted teeth.

"Well"—the twitchy resident looked at the vent screen as if it were in a foreign language—"we usually wait for respiratory therapy to do this. I've never actually run a vent."

"Okay! New plan!" said Jazlyn without skipping a beat. "Don't touch the vent settings. I'll disconnect the tubing and you hold it until I ask for it back. The machine is going to beep because it's disconnected. Just ignore it."

The resident nodded her assent. All eyes were on Dr. Bacani. The room was hers. She took a deep breath and exhaled slowly.

"Disconnecting the vent," she said definitively.

She worked quickly and confidently. After handing off the vent tubing to the resident, she removed the small trach tube, suctioned mucus from the tracheostomy hole, reached for the new trach tube, and attempted to push it into the hole.

No dice.

She tried again, nearly jumping in the air to garner enough force to push the tube in. Still nothing. I took a quick glance at the oxygen saturation: 91 percent. The old lady was coming down pretty quickly. I betrayed no urgency, however. This was Jazzy's show, and she was proving herself a capable director.

"Wow, this scar is tight." She stopped pushing and handed the trach tube back to Ambrosio. She paused for a moment, staring at the hole in the old lady's neck, then suddenly held out her hand again, this time to me. "Lidocaine with epinephrine, Dr. Chin-Quee."

Excellent. It was already in my hand ready to go.

"The uh, the oxygen saturation is down to eighty-nine percent," said the nervous resident.

"Yes, thank you, I'm aware," replied Jazlyn as she injected medication into the skin just below the neck hole. "Fifteen blade."

There you go. I placed the scalpel in her hand, and she quickly made a cut into the scarred skin of the tracheostomy. A little bit of bleeding, but not much. Excellent. *Keep going.*

"Nasal speculum," she said, placing the scalpel on a nearby towel. The speculum was already in my hand, and I handed it over under Ambrosio's incredulous gaze. I spared a glance at him and shrugged. *I guess she has a plan for this.*

A nasal speculum is a small metal tool we use to stretch nostrils when we want to look inside a nose. Though we were dealing with a different hole in the body, Jazlyn would be repurposing it to similar effect. She placed the speculum into the neck hole and squeezed it hard. A few more drops of blood appeared as the hole stretched to a wider diameter. As she removed the speculum a quick *psst psst* escaped her lips and Ambrosio looked up to catch her eye. Jazlyn pouted her lips toward the larger trach in his hand, and Ambrosio handed it over quickly. She pushed with all of the weight of her upper body and the tube, after two stubborn seconds, slipped into the old lady's trachea.

"I'll take the circuit," she said, not looking up from her work space. Dr. Anxiety McTremors handed the vent tubing over to Jazlyn, who connected it to the trach tube. She inflated the tube's cuff with air, and we waited.

Within seconds, the oxygen saturation began to climb. Jazlyn looked at me, bursting with excitement. I returned the glance, imploring her to play it cool. She nodded.

"Okay, so she should be good. There may be a little bit of bleeding from where I made the cut, so place a gauze pad there if needed. You can call us with any questions."

Resident McShaky nodded quickly. Jazlyn strode toward the curtain, paused, turned her head to acknowledge Ambrosio. She smiled and gave a quick nod.

Ambrosio smiled back, his crow's feet and laugh lines betraying the age of his baby face. "Nice job, Doctor," he said.

I closed the tackle box and followed Jazz back into the hallway. She was waiting at the nurse's station, bouncing on her heels.

"Oh my God, you were right!" she squealed. "It feels so much better when your people see you be a fucking *boss*. I had to smile, though. Filipinos have to smile. It's a thing."

"How'd you know he was Filipino?"

"Oh, come on, bro. Asian dude named Ambrosio?"

"Fair enough. Come on, let's go get cookies."

We strolled out of the ER with Jazlyn in the lead, head held high.

"Hey," she said, turning to me, "did you see me not call that resident a fucking idiot?"

I laughed. "I'll be real: I thought you were gonna say something way worse. But honestly, she looked like she was having herself a tough day. You probably just made a new friend."

"Ha ha, yeah, right."

"Hey, you're smart, you're capable, and you're not an asshole. And you had a win today," I said as we turned a corner. "Who *wouldn't* want to be your new friend?"

She nodded to herself for a few silent moments.

"Thanks, Tony," she said.

And off we went to eat empty carbs.

WALDO

"Hey, man. So I ask this with all requisite patience and compassion, but where the fuck is Waldo?"

I closed my eyes in exasperation as Dr. Warovski's nasal Minnesota drawl squawked through the phone speaker. Papers strewn about my resident room desk, a collage of incomplete notes on the computer screen before me, a half-eaten Subway sandwich on my lap. *I didn't have time for this shit right now.*

"Hey, Dr. Warovski. He had to see a consult before scrubbing in with you, so he should be there shortly."

"What time did rounds end this morning?" Dr. Warovski asked, requisite patience out the door.

"Seven fifteen."

"And what kind of consult was it?"

"A trach."

"The current time, according to Steve Jobs's pocket supercomputer, is 9:02 a.m. Am I to believe that it is taking a second-year resident one hour and forty-seven minutes and counting to perform a routine consult on a patient who can't even speak due to the breathing tube in their throat?"

I stifled a smile at this merciless takedown, the precision of which was, dare I say, surgical?

"I guess, yes?" I ventured.

"Very troubling. You need to get your house in order, chief resident."

"Right you are, sir."

"Anyway, this thyroid is taking a bit longer than planned without the assistance of Dr. Waldo, and I've got a patient sitting in clinic who's threatening to burn the place down if she has to wait one more minute to see me. Are you comfortable with coming down and dissecting out the nerve on your own while I hop up and see her?"

An admonishment about my leadership skills immediately followed by a major vote of confidence in my surgical prowess? Fuck it, that was a win in my book. Today was going to be a good day.

"Absolutely. Be down in five."

It had taken a long, long time, but I'd finally reached the residency milestone at which my bosses felt I was safe enough to perform large chunks of operations on my own. And it felt—to use the medical term—dope as fuck. As soon as I'd scrubbed in and

Dr. Warovski had hustled out, I got to work with an assured calm I didn't know I was capable of. The surgical field yawned wide before my eyes, and with the assistance of my battle-tested scrub nurse Sheila, I found in five minutes the nerve that had eluded my attending for thirty.

"Ayyyy, that's a flex. I see you growing up, Chin-Quee," chimed a jovial Sheila.

"Must be the playlist," I said. "Good things happen when I'm finally in charge of the music in here."

"Truth. I've made *all kinds* of things happen in my lifetime when that Boyz II Men comes on."

I laughed. "TMI, inappropriate, and sort of gross, Sheila. But I appreciate the sentiment, so thank you."

She placed a clamp in my hand, didn't let go when I grasped. We locked brown eyes.

"Hey," she said. And then, fully enunciating through her mask in an Arkansas drawl: "We been watching. And we all proud of you."

We. The *we* that was all of us who had seen this world chew up our brown-skinned kind and spit us out.

I nodded and let my eyes do the talking above my mask, finally allowing myself to accept that maybe *we* hadn't been totally misguided in putting faith in *me*.

Of course, faith is nothing if it's never tested. And as I turned my attention back to the surgical bed, the latest test came panting through the OR doors.

Waldo bounded into the room with the grace of a newborn calf—all limbs and a hilarious lack of spatial awareness. Through giggled apologies, he clanged, slipped, and bumped his way to

Sheila's side. As she expertly gowned and gloved him, she shot me another loaded look beneath raised eyebrows: *You'd better come get your boy.*

The only other nonwhite male resident in my program and, despite his having been there only one year, everyone in the hospital seemed to have already decided to give Waldo a wide berth, as if his clumsiness and poor performance were contagious.

Waldo's eyes went wide as he took in the neck wound. "Woah, looks awesome, chief! And Dr. Warovski let you take over for him? So cool!"

"It is indeed highly cool. But I've got to tell you, he was not happy that you never showed up to assist him this morning."

Waldo's demeanor swung dramatically from wonder to contrition. "Yeah. Oh, man, I'm so sorry. I was trying my best to get here, but I wanted to be thorough with my consult, just like you guys have been telling me. And the patient is a good candidate for surgery."

"How long did you spend on the consult?"

Waldo's eyebrows crunched together comically. "Hm. Probably an hour?"

Way too long, especially for a resident who'd done at least twenty similar consults in the last month. Maybe I could offer the benefit of the doubt that he'd indeed spent his time being "thorough."

"Did you get consent from the family?"

"Oh, no, visitor hours haven't started yet."

His earnest puppy-dog eyes belied the absurdity of his words. I cocked my head and asked the obvious question.

"You didn't try to contact them by using any sort of telephone device?"

Waldo's eyebrows shot up, gobsmacked. "Oh! Shoot, no, I didn't think about that."

The fuck? Forget thinking two steps ahead, this kid didn't even know what a step was. Okay, that was mean. More benefit-of-the-doubt time. Come on, Waldo, redeem your goddamn self.

"And did you put the patient on the surgery schedule for tomorrow?" I asked.

"Not yet. I know that should be the next step, so I'll do it as soon as we finish up here."

Swing and a miss. And the guy had no idea how widely he was missing.

"Okay, just so I'm clear," I began, straining for a light glaze of patience and compassion, "it took one hour to do a history and physical on an unconscious patient, and in that time you didn't complete all of the consult tasks and left them for someone else to do?"

"No no no!" Waldo recoiled, thoroughly scandalized. Sheila grabbed hold of the suction tool in his hand, as his errant movement had nearly put a blood vessel at risk. What a fucking pro. Waldo went on, oblivious, "I'm totally going to get them done as soon as we're done operating!"

"No, Waldo, you've been on call all night, so after we finish operating, you're going home so that you don't violate duty hours."

His shoulders slumped, all vigor suddenly sapped. "You're right," he said softly. "I'm sorry."

I regarded him curiously, unnerved by his cartoonishly exaggerated mood swings. There was something strange about young Dr. Waldo. I turned my attention back to the operation, venturing one last question in the name of completeness.

"So what else did you get into after the consult?"

"I just ran to get a quick breakfast," he said. Then, off my expectant, over-the-rims-of-my-hipster-framed-glasses look, he admitted, "And went to the bathroom."

"Took another hour, huh?"

Eyes downcast. "Yeah."

If Waldo was to be believed, he'd had the longest bowl of Cheerios ever followed by the most epic shit of his life. And I wasn't sure that I did believe him. And that was a problem.

As if she could read my thoughts, Sheila slipped me a side-eyed glance: *This poor chile slippin'*.

"Hey, man, listen," I began as I refocused on peeling the thyroid gland away from the trachea, "I know it seems like you're always playing catch-up, and in certain respects that's a part of the job that will never go away. But the bosses are already talking about you, and that's never a good thing as a second-year. They should barely know your name. But since they do, we should work on a rebranding campaign, know what I mean?"

In response, Waldo's suction tool drifted slowly toward my beautifully dissected nerve, threatening to paralyze it. I swatted it quickly out of harm's way and raised my head to find Waldo asleep on his feet, head lolling to his gown. Jeez. Personality weirdness aside, I knew I'd been where he was—always one step behind, struggling to anticipate what was expected, and always, always dangerously tired. Time for an intervention.

"Waldo," I ventured forcefully. Nothing. I looked to Sheila, who nodded, removed all tools from his sagging hands, stepped back from the table, and clapped her palms together in a percussive blast just inches from Waldo's left ear.

"Oh God!" Waldo's head snapped up, eyes wild.

"Morning, sunshine," I said.

"I'm sorry I . . . no, I just . . . What was the question?"

"No question, Waldo. You're sleepwalking and that's not safe. I'm sending you home. Go sleep, please."

He made to argue but I just shook my head. "Trust me. When someone sends you home to sleep, don't argue. Just meet me before rounds tomorrow morning. I want to touch base about how you're doing."

Without another word, he pulled off his gown and gloves and slipped out of the room. Sheila slapped a scissor into my palm.

"It's tough being grown, huh?" she asked, organizing her tray of instruments. "Before you know it, the kids are giving you white whiskers."

I nodded. "I'm just trying to gray gracefully."

"Good luck with that plan, Doc."

K obe!"

The empty cup from which I'd just slurped the remnants of a smoothie rolled from my fingertips. Perfect hook-shot form. The cup sailed across the tiny office, banked off the wall and into a trash bin.

I pumped my fist, stretched, and rubbed the dregs of sleep from my eyes. "Damn, Chin-Quee, how you so multitalented?" I asked aloud. Another minute ticked by on the wall clock: 6:18 a.m. I'd been waiting for Waldo for eighteen long minutes. His exclamatory texts over the last few minutes were riddled with falsehoods of the most transparent variety:

Sorry, blocked in by the garbage truck!!

Accident at the freeway on-ramp!!

> 5 min away!
>
> Sad emoji!
>
> Parking now!

Bitch, you overslept. Own your slipups like a grown-up.

As entertained as I'm generally able to keep myself in solitude, this shit was getting ridiculous. 6:20 a.m. Where the fuck was—

"Oh, man, chief, I'm so sorry!" Waldo came panting through the door of the bare spare office with the maniacally genial countenance of a Muppet.

"It seems like you're always out of breath any time you arrive anywhere." I pushed a chair his way as he pulled off his down jacket.

"Yeah, I know." His eyes darkened for a blink of a moment, then a toothy grin. "Seems like the only way I can make it to all of the places I'm supposed to be is if I'm running!"

He laughed nervously, eyebrows pleading with me to join in. Instead I reached for my phone and pulled up an email: a list from the General of all of the gripes against Waldo that had been circulating among the attendings. I'd learned since my days as a junior resident that these sorts of gripes, though completely unhelpful in improving performance, would fester in the minds of the bosses and threaten to derail any hope of earning their trust as the years went on.

But as a senior resident, this was my house. I had to defend it.[2] I'd had to navigate the same bullshit on my own a couple of years earlier, but as weird as Waldo was, he deserved a better chance to succeed. And step one of that plan was to translate a list of disgruntled complaints into constructive feedback.

---

2. Shout-out to Kevin McCallister, circa 1990.

"Waldo, we're pressed for time, so I'm just going to jump in. The bosses are . . . concerned with your performance so far."

"Oh no!" Waldo's eyebrows shot up in disbelief.

"Oh yes," I continued, taking a moment to study his response. *Is he seriously surprised by this news?* "But it's okay. I struggled when I started on service too. It's a strange world with strange demands, and I know you're doing the best you can. I thought it might help to demystify the expectations with you and see what we can do about getting you up to speed."

"Thank you. Thank you so much for taking the time, chief. I appreciate it so much. I know I can do this. I will do this." His head nodded fervently as his gaze fell to the carpet. Then, to himself, "I *will* do this."

I took a look at my list: *(1) Waldo is late to everything. We can't rely on him to be on time for AM rounds, or any assignments in the OR or clinic. He's never where we need him to be.* Oof. Okay, here goes.

"So, we've noticed that you have trouble getting places on time. Happens to the best of us, and I know it's not purposeful. But let's start with the mornings. How about you schedule your morning routines as if rounds start at six fifteen instead of six thirty. Give yourself some buffer time in case, you know, you're ever blocked in by the garbage truck again."

"That's really good advice, chief. Really good. Yeah, I'll definitely do that. I totally have trouble getting up and going in the morning, so I'll do better."

"How many alarms do you set in the morning?"

"Oh, just the one. But I will admit I usually hit snooze a couple of times, hahahaha."

Weird thing to laugh about, bro.

"Here's a quick fix," I said. "Set no fewer than three alarms, three or four minutes apart. You can't snooze them all because they keep coming at you."

Waldo went slack-jawed, as if I'd just dazzled him with close-up magic. "Ohhhhhhh. Of course, why didn't I think of that? You're a genius! Nice!"

Back to the list: *(2) Waldo gets tasks done either incompletely or not at all. His forgetfulness is quickly approaching unacceptable levels.* Sheesh. No veil of subtext here: the bosses were *not* happy with my man Waldo. I could still work with it, however. Beneath the unnecessary snark, the through line of the first two complaints on this list was—

"Okay, next up I want to talk about organization and time management. I've noticed that you've been having some trouble with getting assignments done completely and in a decent time frame. What's your system for keeping your to-do list organized each day?"

"Oh! I just try to do it the way I've seen everyone else do it," said Waldo as he rummaged through his messenger bag. "I just write things down on my list so that—ah! Here it is! Ta-da!"

He handed me a piece of paper that was nearly weighed down by the amount of ink on both sides. In the white space around and between each patient's typed description were countless inscrutable notes written in Waldo's tightly coiled, minuscule cursive. My eyes nearly crossed as I tried to decipher the scrawled writing, prompting another silly-ass giggle from Waldo.

"I know, I write small! Actually, that's a little smaller than normal, just because I want to make sure I fit everything on the page. I swear, I write down everything I'm told to do. It's all there."

"Even if it's all there, it's no help if you can't see it."

"I can see it," shot Waldo, suddenly intense. "I can read all of it. I'm not . . ."

His eyes fell to the floor again as he suddenly lost himself in thought. But only for a moment. In an instant, his eyes came back into focus. He looked to his hands, found them clenched, and quickly released his fingers. Before I knew it, his million-dollar smile was on display once again.

"Everything's there, chief."

"I know everything's there," I said, searching his eyes. I wasn't sure what was going on behind that smile, but my instincts told me that validation was a good idea at this moment. "But even so, you might be making your life harder than it needs to be. Look, back in high school, calculus kicked my ass for weeks and I couldn't figure out why. I knew the shit in class, but I'd always get the problems wrong on my homework. Turns out it was because I was writing everything too small, trying to save space. I made my own writing too hard to follow and ended up missing stuff."

Waldo's smile remained plastered on, but I couldn't shake the feeling that a shadow had passed before his eyes at the mention of high school. No matter. Keep going.

"What I'm saying is," I continued, "it might do you good to give yourself some more space. Staple a blank page to your list in the morning. Jack up that font size on your writing. You're spending your days tired and hungry. Make that one thing easier on yourself."

Waldo nodded. And kept nodding. Smiling and nodding. All in silence. The fuck was going on here?

"And regarding time management," I went on, "that's something I and the other seniors should be better about helping you with. You get a million phone calls a day, feel like you're being pulled in a million different directions. It's totally over-whelming. So we'll do our best to help you prioritize your tasks so that you end up being where you need to be on time throughout the day."

"Yes, thanks, thanks, thank you," Waldo sputtered. "Your help would be really . . . Yeah, thank you."

Time to wrap this up. Something about this interaction was . . . I wasn't even sure, but I very much wanted to get out of that room. I scrolled down to the last item on the list: *(3) Waldo doesn't know what he doesn't know.*

I met Waldo's gaze once more. His smiling eyes danced in an uncanny intersection of ecstasy, desperation, and mania. They held me transfixed as I contemplated the gravity of this last complaint. When it came to patient interactions, Waldo carried himself with an unearned hubris. On multiple occasions he'd given patients in-correct diagnoses, ordered incorrect medications at incorrect dos-ages, and even performed minor procedures when they weren't indicated. It's not unusual to give off a bit of an air of unearned confidence—that's just part of the job of a medical trainee—but to be unaware of your limitations? That's where young doctors be-come dangerous. And Waldo's rogue inclinations had set him on a path to becoming very, very dangerous.

I had no idea how to course-correct the young doctor seated before me. The fact that Waldo felt he could intuit his way to a diagnosis and through a treatment plan bolstered only by his beginner-level knowledge of medicine was baked into some key-stone of his personality. It wasn't something I could fix in my lim-ited chief resident capacity. All I could do was hope that he got there on his own, and keep as many people safe as I could by look-ing over his shoulder.

"Last thing, then I'll let you go." I leaned forward. Waldo teetered on the edge of his seat. "Our main goal here is that we all become safe doctors. That's why we train. Nobody expects you to know every answer right out of the gate, so we expect you to ask lots of questions at this stage. You tend not to ask questions often enough, and sometimes that lands you in trouble. So starting today, I expect you to run your assessment and plan by a senior resident as soon as you complete a consult so that we can make sure we're all on the same page."

Waldo's lips curled. Just a bit. The slightest hint of a sneer.

"Every consult? Even the simple ones?"

I nodded. "Every single consult."

"It just seems a bit like . . ." Waldo waved his hands through the air, searching for words, pleading with his eyes. "Chief, I know I can do this. I get that I've got to make some tweaks and improvements, and I swear I'll make them happen. Swear on my mother. But this is all starting to feel like nobody trusts me."

"That's because you're right. Nobody trusts you."

I let the truth hang in the air as Waldo's irises shook in his eye sockets with well-concealed contempt. Fuck the good cop routine. I'd had enough.

"Here's what I need you to understand. I want you to succeed. I believe that you can. But you've got a mountain to climb, because a bunch of the bosses are *this* close to giving up on you. All of the issues we've been talking about? They're coming straight from the top. And what's more, they've requested that we start documenting any time you slip up. You understand what that means?"

Waldo's face morphed into a caricature of dread. He knew what that shit meant.

"It means that they're gathering evidence so that they can be justified in putting you on probation, or even holding you back a year. This shit is serious, man."

Waldo's eyes wandered the room, vacant. His lips quivered, whispering words only he could hear.

"Your job this month is to help me make my report on you as short and innocuous as possible."

"Yes, sir," said Waldo, nearly inaudibly.

"Okay. Why don't you head over for rounds?"

Waldo gathered his things and, head down, made for the door.

"Hey." I put a hand on his shoulder, stilling him. "You can do this."

He gave a noncommittal nod and walked into the hallway, closing the door behind him.

I pocketed my phone and deflated with a heaving sigh into my chair, kicked off my Danksos, and let my head flop back. I was troubled. Big time. By that point in my life I'd negotiated plenty of challenging feedback sessions, both as the feedbackee and the feedbacker, but this was the first time I'd left one with the overwhelming need to take a shower—like, a super hot one with industrial disinfectant–grade soap and a pumice stone. Interacting with Waldo just made me feel gross. And I didn't know why. By all accounts, I should have been bubbling over with empathy for the guy: brown-skinned kid in medicine; underperforming and overtired; struggling to adhere to rules both written and unwritten; shouldering the heavy weight of low expectations; wearing a carefully constructed mask to keep his struggles hidden. I knew it all so intimately. Many of the bruises from my fight were still ripe, the gashes still raw. Now I had a front-row seat to Waldo's battle royale, and he was taking a bloody beating.

And yet it was his mask that rattled me. It was the plastered smile and the wild laughter. It was the goofy parlance and the Looney Tunes facial expressions. It was the unsustainable eye contact and the micro mood swings. It was the lack of self-awareness of his jarring moments of pride and anger and confidence and doubt.

And there it was: *Waldo had no idea he was even wearing a mask.*

What's more, his mask was under attack—mercilessly hammered, cracked, and broken bit by bit with each passing day in the hospital. His protective shell was falling away in massive chunks and he was completely oblivious. Not only that, I had the distinct notion that beneath his failing veil lay a visage he neither knew nor understood. He'd soon come face-to-face with the man he'd been hiding from himself, and, given the instability he'd exuded to this point, it was likely he wouldn't like what he saw. That clash could prove dark. Or dangerous. And I had no confidence that it wouldn't happen right there in the hospital. Possibly in front of his coworkers. Or worse yet, a patient.

Where's Waldo, indeed.

Okay. The race card. I'm officially playing the race card."

Ira pushed his chair back from his computer and cast his eyes around the resident room in search of an audience. No response but the continued clicks of fingertips on keyboards. He doubled down.

"It's Yom Kippur, arguably the holiest of High Holidays, and not only am I forced to work, but the cafeteria doesn't even commemorate the occasion with matzo ball soup. Racist."

Jazlyn clicked a baby carrot between her teeth and rolled her eyes deep into the back of her head. "It's not racist because Jews aren't a race."

"Fuck that," Ira spat emphatically. "Race is a social construct. And *society* has been *constructed* to hate and starve out my people since the Old Testament."

"You know what's actually racist is that goddamn soup," Jazlyn said between bites. "It's so fucking bland, and the matzo balls taste like doughy ass. Eating it sucks and borders on a hate crime against *me*."

Ira, thoroughly scandalized and dismayed, leaned back to study Jazzy with pity. "My God, who hurt you?"

Jazz, mouth full of carrot, shot back, "Why are you the way you are?"

"Fuck off."

"Eat a dick!"

"Oh my God, can you two at least pretend like you have work to do?" I pleaded, eyes on my computer screen.

Jazlyn insolently snapped another carrot, prompting me to shut my eyes in an urgent call for serenity. A pall of anxiety hung thick in the resident room these days. Jazlyn and Ira's sibling-like ribbing had become progressively more barbed and mean-spirited, and I had long since lost the bandwidth to referee them. I turned to check on Yumi, the most junior resident in the room, and found her silently scribbling notes as she clicked through patient charts on a screen. She'd grown quieter over the last few weeks, taking up as little space as possible as the demands on her time ratcheted up. Yumi was a second-year and, tragically, Waldo's coresident. His mistakes were her extra work, which she completed correctly and without complaint. But a passing glance at her bloodshot eyes and tightly drawn mouth painted a picture of a woman who couldn't keep this up for much longer.

I wanted so badly to prioritize the sanity and well-being of my cherished crew of uniquely weird young ENT surgeons, but the events outlined on the screen before me had monopolized every bit of my spare time and energy for the last month:

> **9/3:** Waldo printed out the daily patient list late. The list was incomplete, no updated labs or vitals. We learned once we reached an ICU patient's room that they'd had a critically low hemoglobin value last night and were in need of a blood transfusion, however they could not get the transfusion order from Waldo because he never answered the multiple pages they sent him.
>
> **9/6:** During this morning's educational conference, the residents were given a five-minute break in between sessions. Waldo left and returned 20–30 min later with a tray of breakfast. He missed half of our guest lecturer's presentation.
>
> **9/10:** Last night, Waldo was called to evaluate an urgent airway. He saw the patient and recommended admission to the ICU. However, Waldo never wrote down the patient's name or medical record number, so we spent rounds this morning searching for the patient based on his admit floor and ethnicity. Once we found the patient, we performed an airway exam and found that Waldo's description of the exam was inaccurate. The patient should never have been admitted to the hospital in the first place.

The list went on and on.

I looked at the time and shook my head: 6:42 a.m. Waldo had been on call the night before, so we couldn't start rounds without him. Twelve minutes late and counting.

"Can someone page him, please?" I asked the room, rubbing the tension out of my jaw muscles with my fingertips. Without a word, Yumi's fingers flew over the keypad of the nearest phone, shooting an urgent message to Waldo's hip somewhere in the hospital.

Three seconds later, the familiar chirps of a pager erupted to my left. Jazlyn dropped her carrots, rummaged through a pile of loose desk papers, and let out an astonished "You've got to be fucking kidding me."

Mouth agape, she lifted Waldo's pager from the clutter for all to see. Ira erupted in laughter. "Oh my God, that's so fucking classic."

Hair fell over Yumi's eyes as her head dropped to her chest, despondent.

Fucking hell. By the minute Waldo was inventing new ways to prove himself inept. Ira's hands grabbed hold of my shoulders from behind and began massaging.

"Damn, is that the shit list?" Ira scanned the mess of entries on my screen. "Let me give you some icing on this turd cake. So I ran into some buddies who work at the hospital where Waldo went to med school, and when I told them that he'd matched with us, know what they did? They *laughed.* For, like, an uncomfortable amount of time."

I sighed and scratched at my beard scruff.

"I mean, what the fuck?" Ira went on. "How many times has this kid been pushed through to the next stage even though the whole world knew he was trash? How does that help *him*?"

And with that dubious cue, Turd Cake himself burst through the door.

"Sorry, sorry, I know," muttered Waldo flatly as he handed out copies of the patient list.

"Forget something?" Jazlyn asked, holding up Waldo's pager.

"Oh, yeah, that's mine." Waldo chuckled, forcing a smile through chapped lips.

"Waldo, we always need to be able to find you," I said, scanning the freshly copied pages before me. "That means the pager has to stay on your hip. Like, at all times."

I caught his eyes from across the room. He nodded and took a seat. And kept sitting. In glazed-eye silence.

"Whenever you're ready," I said forcefully, prompting Waldo's face to jerk back to life. The rest of the residents shared sideways glances across the room.

"Right!" Waldo's energy shot back up to 100 percent. He ran a confident hand through his disheveled mop of hair. "Okay, so Mr. Fariq, post-op day one from a tracheostomy. I got called for some bleeding from the site last night, so I placed some pieces of Surgicel in the wound and he did well after that."

Yumi's brow furrowed. Ira massaged his nasal bridge. Jazlyn snapped a carrot and looked to me with wide eyes.

Goddamn it, Waldo.

"Waldo," I began, straining mightily for patience, "can you think of any reason why placing a bunch of tiny, loose pieces of fabric into someone's trach wound might be a bad idea?"

"Well, no? I mean, it stopped the bleeding."

"You placed a bunch of small foreign bodies into a hole that leads directly into the trachea. One sharp inhalation or change in body position and that stuff flies straight into his lungs. Respiratory failure. Not great. I know you've never seen any of us stop trach bleeding that way. That's why I need you to call your senior before you act."

Waldo's jaw clenched beneath his sallow cheeks.

"Yumi, you and I will go right after rounds to remove as much as we can." Yumi's pen scratched the plan quickly onto a notepad. I turned back to Waldo. "Next patient."

"Okay, Ms. DeVille, post-op day one after melanoma excision and scalp reconstruction, did well overnight, pain controlled, tolerating a diet."

"Woah." Ira dramatically pulled his patient list to within three inches of his eyeballs. "Those scalp drain outputs are super high. Were they collecting a lot of blood?"

"They were initially, so I set all of the drains to wall suction so that blood wouldn't collect under the scalp."

Ira jumped in before I had the chance. "So I'm assuming you don't find anything wrong with that plan?"

"It would appear that I don't," Waldo growled through gritted teeth.

"When you connect those drains to mechanical wall suction, you remove blood faster, yes, but the force of the suction causes the scalp to heal unevenly. The space under the scalp gets walled off like a honeycomb and provides lots of fun spots for infections to hide." Ira squeezed his face between his palms in frustration. "Fuck, dude, the General's gonna rip our assholes out through our earholes when he finds out. Waldo, man, you're not at the level where you can just change treatment plans overnight."

"Yeah, but did she die?" muttered Waldo under his breath.

"What?" asked Ira, even though we all knew what we'd just heard.

"Next patient," said Waldo. Ira turned to me, mouthing an irritated *The fuck?* Jazlyn stared intently at her computer screen, willing herself not to laugh at the mounting absurdity. Yumi scribbled notes silently.

"Ms. Dorian, post-op day one after a tracheostomy yesterday,"

Waldo pushed on with wooden resolve. "I performed a thorough exam on her last night and noted evidence of subcutaneous air in her neck tissue. So I grabbed an ultrasound machine and performed a needle aspiration of several small air pockets."

Stunned silence. I probed my mind for any justification Waldo could give me for performing this batshit procedure, found none, felt pressure suddenly rise behind my eyes, and lost the last precious remnants of my chill.

"What?" I left *the fucking fuck* off the end of my exclamation in a last-ditch nod to professionalism.

Waldo looked back at me as if I were the fucking crazy one. "The indication was air in the neck tissue. It could have been an early indication of a deep neck space infection."

"Was there any evidence of infection?" I went in. Hard. "Was the neck red, hot, and inflamed? Pus draining? Fever? White count?"

"Not, uh, that I could see."

"The answer to those questions is 'no.' And even if there was an infection as the root cause, we treat the infection because the air bubbles in neck tissue won't kill anybody. But a series of needle pokes into the deep neck by a second-year resident might. Would you agree?"

Waldo's body went rigid as I picked apart his logic. He managed a stiff nod of his head.

"And finally," I continued, "can you think of any other highly reasonable explanation as to why Ms. Dorian might have air bubbles in her neck?"

Everyone had gone still in the resident room. Though I was straining for educational decorum, the fact that Waldo's overnight adventures had put two patients at risk of serious illness and fucking *death* left me stripped of all patience and compassion. I was ready to yell, scream, or throw something small and dense, but I found myself stayed by the wary stares of my junior residents just as I was about to tip over the edge. I was the leader of this team, and my team deserved a leader who wouldn't be goaded into histrionics with every act of supreme foolishness.

"No guesses?" I resumed with measured volume and tone. "The answer is her tracheostomy operation, aka that time yesterday afternoon when we cut a big-ass fucking hole into her neck through which she now breathes pressurized air every three seconds."

Okay, so I wasn't going to win the Richard Roundtree Smoothest and Least Profane Dude in a Roomful of Constant Bullshit Award, but I tried. Still, it wasn't enough to stop Jazlyn from snorting a chuckle under her breath.

Waldo's weary eyes sharpened in an instant and shot daggers into the back of Jazlyn's head. Every muscle from his neck down tensed with such ferocity that I could practically hear them buzzing. His patient list crinkled softly as he sawed through the paper with his fingernails.

Something had finally snapped inside Waldo. He was no longer with us. His eyes were wild, his body alight with the savage desperation of a stray dog.

Shit. He was going to take Jazlyn's fucking head off.

He shifted in his seat, threatening to rise. I shifted in my own, ready to meet him, when—

Beebeebeep! Beebeebeep!

Waldo's pager chimed out, defusing the charged silence. He sprang from his seat and swiped it violently from Jazlyn's desk as she flinched in surprise.

"I'm gonna answer that," spat Waldo as he flung open a storage cabinet and began chucking papers, pens, and pocket instruments into it with clanging abandon. Then, rounding on me, "They've always got to be able to find me, right?"

He threw the cabinet door closed with a crash, jolting the other residents into their seat backs with the shock wave.

All right, fuck this shit. I stood up, infinitely grateful that I stood several inches taller than my unstable coworker.

"Okay, Waldo, you and I are going to have a chat outside. Right now. Let's go."

Waldo wasted no time and was out the door before I'd finished speaking. "You guys finish running the list," I continued to the troops. "I'll catch up."

Jazlyn mouthed a wide-eyed and sheepish *I'm sorry* as I made my way to the door. I shook my head and shrugged in defeat. *No, I'm sorry.*

I found Waldo in a tiny office across the hall, pacing in tight circles. I closed the door behind me.

"You got something you need to say?"

"I'm just . . . just . . ." Waldo's arms flailed before him, grasping for invisible purchase. "I'm sick of this shit! And Jazz. Jazz, she's always just waiting, you know? Just waiting for me to screw up, and if I do, she fucking loves it. Just can't wait to stick it to me and laugh in my face."

"I'll talk to her," I said evenly. "It was not okay for her to laugh, though I don't think it was malicious. It might be one of the ways she reacts when she's uncomfortable."

Waldo pinned his eyes on me while his body continued its frantic march. "Give me a break, Tony. She's out to get me. *All of you* are out to get me. I'm giving this job everything I have. More than everything. And everyone just shits on me until I have nothing left!"

He came to a stop and sat on the edge of a nearby desk, head buried in his hands, fingers writhing and clawing in his hair. "I know you already know about what happened this weekend with the patient who didn't get their transfusion. Dr. Warovski chewed me out on rounds that morning for like twenty minutes. Just ripped me apart. And afterwards I went to my car and—" He lifted his face from his hands and looked to the ceiling. "Look, I never cry. It's just not a thing I do. I didn't even cry at my brother's funeral. But I sat in my car this weekend and I cried harder than I ever have in my entire life. *That's* how much I'm giving to this. That's how much all of you are taking away from me!"

Waldo's leg shot out, connected with a trash bin. It sailed across the tiny space, crashed into the adjacent desk, and sent garbage flying.

Well, shit. This situation was officially fucked. The real Waldo had finally emerged, and he was even more unstable than I'd thought possible. Unpacking his paranoia, rage, and grief-processing issues was the job of some saintly future therapist. Right now, *my* job was simpler: defuse this eruption and get the fuck out of this tiny room in one piece.

"Waldo," I said, choosing my words slowly and carefully, "I hear you. I hear your anger and your frustration. I know that you are doing your best, and I understand—"

"Oh, stop acting like you give a shit about me. You don't care about how I feel or what I'm going through, so just fucking spare me." Waldo was on his feet again, stepping toward me. "I'm not stupid. I hear all of the big sighs, I see all the secret looks flying around the room. I know you're all always talking shit about me before I walk into the room and as soon as I leave. And you . . ."

He took another step closer, stuck a finger in my face. One inch from my nose. Saliva sprayed on my cheeks with each word.

"I know you think I'm dumb. It's in the way you talk to me and I fucking hate it, so fuck you and your condescending bullshit!"

What *should* have happened is twofold.

First, the entire room should have shaken with the sound of the back of my hand leaving a five-fingered, bone-deep mark of remembrance on the side of Waldo's unstable-ass head.

Second, Waldo's head should have subsequently fallen neatly into the aforementioned trash bin and crunched pathetically against soiled napkins and coffee cups.

Because what the fuck was this motherfucker thinking? Spitting in my face, finger an inch from my eye, screaming at the top of his lungs?

In Detroit, motherfuckers get sent to the emergency room for *far* less.

It took every ounce of self-control to quell my raging hoodstincts. Consequences, I reminded myself, were a sad reality. If ever I were to be arrested for assault and battery, it wasn't going to be over *fucking Waldo*.

I opted instead for the power of silence. That and the summoning of my best Lauryn Hill–at–the–end–of–*Sister Act 2*—when–she's–about–to–sing–"Joyful Joyful"–at–the–choir–championships–but–her–mother–who–didn't–want–her–to–sing–shows–up–and–they–lock–eyes–and–delay–the–start–of–the–song withering gaze. I held Waldo's eyes in a vise grip. Unblinking. Daring him to make a final foolish decision.

Silent seconds passed. He slowly lowered his finger.

"Here's what you need to know," I began softly, forcing him to be quiet enough to listen. "My responsibility is not to you. It's not even to the other residents. My primary responsibility, above all else, is to keep our patients alive and safe. In order to do that, I have to make sure each of us is a safe doctor. And right now, you are not safe to be around patients."

Waldo's eyes bored into me, jaw muscles quivering.

"You need to go home, Waldo."

"No," he scoffed, feet pacing once again. "No, I don't. I have work to finish and I'm going to get it done."

"No, you are not. Listen to me." I waited for my silence to still his steps. "You are literally kicking and screaming in a clinic office. This room is not soundproofed. You haven't had the presence of mind to process that everything you've been shouting can be heard all the way down the hall. By other doctors. By nurses. And by patients."

The rabid fighting spirit drained from his muscles with each calmly delivered word. He shut his eyes tight and dropped his chin to his chest, as if trying to will away the inevitable.

"Where you're at right now is not okay," I continued, "so you will go home. Right now. We'll figure out what comes next later today."

Without another word, Waldo walked past me to the door and left. I stepped out a moment later and looked down the hallway to find several doors cracked open. Anxious eyes and slack jaws peeked out of the doorways with trepidation.

Shit.

What a mess.

My phone buzzed while I was midbite on some sumptuous-ass Thai food. I looked down, saw the caller, swallowed fast, swigged water, cleared my throat, and hit accept. The Boss was calling.

The Boss was the biggest of our cheeses. Our department chair. My bosses' boss. She spoke fast, moved even faster, and struck fear into the hearts of men—a valuable trait in our male-dominated profession. Plus, I'd heard a rumor that she needed only ninety minutes of sleep a night, which, if true, both terrified and impressed me.

You always answered the Boss on the first ring.

"Hey, Boss," I said, closing my eyes in preparation for the barrage of lightning-quick words I'd be expected to understand the first and only time she said them.

"Hi.So,IheardwhathappenedtodaywithWaldoandIwantedtoget youraccountbeforedecidingonhowtoproceedwithhim."

See? Fast.

I gave her the rundown of our encounter in the tiny office in her preferred style: succinct but with every pertinent detail.

She jumped in as soon as I'd finished. "Fascinating.WellI'mglad you'reallright.Here'smyquestionforyou.You'rechiefresidentsoyou've spentmoretimewithhimthananyoftheseniorstaff.Whatdoyouthink weshoulddowithWaldo?"

As was her wont, the Boss cut right to the heart of the matter. And she was, uncharacteristically, soliciting my opinion. My next words would hold massive weight. I had to make them count.

Even after everything, I empathized with Waldo just as I empathized with all of the residents I'd known who struggled in a system that wasn't built for their success. I knew that I'd done the best I could in my limited capacity to help him navigate this unforgiving world, but ultimately he had failed. He had failed because we'd failed him.

All of us. His peers (myself included) and superiors failed to provide him the type of support he needed to succeed. But greater than that, Waldo was failed by the entirety of the medical education system. He was the shining antithesis to the argument that good grades and book smarts are the main predictors of who will become a great doctor. In this age of ninety-ninth-percentile MCAT and Step and Board scores as entrance keys to the profession, we too often neglect to screen for traits that truly matter: the self-awareness and strength of character necessary to weather the devastating emotional trials that are sure to come; the humility and grace required to be an effective, collaborative, and avid lifelong learner. Perhaps it's because a rigorous evaluation for those characteristics in each applicant would take too much time and effort. Or maybe the decision makers just don't prioritize the humanity, emotional intelligence, and resolve of the next generation. Either way you slice it, the system pushes the Waldos of the world through. He'd had the grades—he was a sure thing. Advancing him was the path of least resistance.

At least until he self-destructed like a dying star, threatening to suck in and destroy everything in his gravitational pull.

So what to do about Waldo?

Maybe it was the last year of hard-fought self-actualization, or maybe it was the Thai food, but either way I was awash not with conflict but with clarity. I owned my part in Waldo's failure, but for once, I didn't internalize it. I felt no temptation to spiral into misguided affirmations that I too was a failure. No need to make myself a martyr by requesting that he get second, third, fifth, and tenth chances as an act of self-flagellation. My only hope was to stop the cascade of failures and extend one last kindness to a young man who still had so much left to find in his life.

"Boss, I think Waldo is going through a tough time right now and should probably consider speaking to a therapist to try and help him get back on track. But if I'm thinking about his fitness more globally, based on what I've seen over the last several months"—I took a breath to steady myself—"I don't think he should be an ENT resident anymore. Here or anywhere."

Silence on the other end of the phone.

"I'm not confident that he should even be in this profession," I said with finality.

"Got it," replied the Boss, with no indication of where her head was at. "You'redoingagreatjobTonyI'llseeyoutomorrowbyebye."

Waldo was placed on indefinite leave that day. Ultimately, he was asked not to return. The residents pulled together—working extra hours, taking extra nights on call—to pick up the slack. Everyone was a little busier, a lot more tired, but the black cloud had lifted and its absence was worth it.

Every morning from then on, just as rounds were set to begin, I'd silently wish Waldo well. And hope that he'd never touch a patient again.

LORISA

4:28 a.m.

I jolted awake, grasping for the singing pager on my nightstand when another chime rang out—text message incoming.

As I felt around in the dark for my phone, it started ringing urgently.

Goddamn. The triple threat. Someone really wanted to chat.

I checked the caller ID and set the hand piece to my ear.

"What up, LoLo," I mumbled, wiping sleep out of my eyelids.

Lorisa's uncharacteristically rapid, pressured speech perked me up immediately. "Hey, Tony, so Mr. Asaad, our robotic radical tonsillectomy guy, started bleeding from the mouth about twenty minutes ago. It's pretty brisk."

I sat bolt upright. Mr. Asaad was a salvage cancer patient—he'd had throat cancer years ago and received chemo and radiation to treat it, then the cancer had returned three months ago in the same place. We'd done an extensive robotic cancer resection on him three days prior, and it had been a nightmare: dissecting through tissue that had been through radiation was like trying to chop wood with a butter knife. The guy was at risk for every complication under the sun.

"Do you need me to come in?"

"Um . . ." Her hesitation didn't inspire confidence. "Well, I tried to get pressure on the bleed, but I couldn't slow it down. Then his sats started dropping, so they're trying to intubate him now and—"

"Lorisa." I could hear the panic rising in my junior resident's voice despite her admirable attempts at calm. "Do you need me to come in?"

"Well, yeah, I think I need some help."

"I'll be there in fifteen. Use a suction to pack strip gauze into his tonsil bed if you can't see through the blood. And do *not* let anyone but an attending attempt to intubate him."

I was at the patient's door in ten.

The room was bloody, alarm-blaring chaos.

ICU residents, anesthesia residents, nurses, respiratory thera-pists, pharmacists, all jockeying for position and shouting orders over Mr. Asaad's stripped, still body.

At the head of the bed stood Lorisa, holding her own as she suctioned blood while speaking rapidly with the anesthesia attend-ing to her left.

I crossed the threshold and took in the vitals: 19 percent oxy-gen in his blood, no heartbeat. Flatline. Sweat poured from a mas-sively muscular nurse's face as he pounded chest compressions. A resident at the foot of the bed shouted for more epinephrine. In response, another nurse shouted, "One milligram epi in at four forty-one." In the breathless turmoil, forgotten in a corner, stood a terrified, stone-still mother and daughter.

I caught a nurse's ear. "Hey, can you please take his family members out of here as quickly as you can? They've already seen too much of this."

She nodded and moved to them while I gloved up and made my way to Lorisa's side.

"He coded as soon as we got off the phone," she said through a blood-spattered face shield. "We haven't been able to get the breathing tube down."

"How many attempts?" I asked the diminutive anesthesia at-tending to my left.

"Five to this point. I can't see the airway through the blood."

"Got it. Can I take a look?" I offered, more a polite demand than a question.

He stepped aside and I grabbed the tools.

"Okay, LoLo, the bleeding is coming from the inferior pole of the tonsillar fossa, so I want you to get some fresh gauze, place it in that spot, and apply pressure up toward the ceiling with your suction."

Lorisa moved quickly, quietly, and correctly. In seconds the bleeding slowed from geyser to kitchen faucet, partially due to Lorisa's quick moves and partially due to the fact that the guy no longer had a heartbeat with which to pump blood. I seized the opportunity to get a good look down his throat, slipped in the breathing tube, and attached an Ambu bag, which I handed off to a waiting nurse. As he began squeezing air into Mr. Asaad's lungs, I stepped away to the side of the bed. Lorisa's ashen face watched the monitors as her arms quivered with the exertion of holding pressure on the bleeder.

I folded my arms and watched the monitor right along with her. Solidarity was important, even when I'd known the man was dead when I walked in the door.

"Hold compressions," shouted the ICU resident. All activity in the room came to a weary halt.

"Time of death: four fifty-five a.m."

I looked to Lorisa, whose haunted eyes were already locked on mine. I motioned with my head for her to meet me outside.

"You have any consults waiting for you?" I asked when we reached the nurses' station.

"Well"—she watched the somber mass exodus from the dead man's room in a detached trance—"a couple of trach consults, foreign body in some kid's ear in the ER . . ."

"Anyone suffocating or bleeding?"

"No," she replied dreamily, "nobody suffocating or . . ."

She was teetering. Shell-shocked.

I knew what she needed.

"Hey," I said. She snapped back to life and turned in the

direction of my voice. "Fuck that kid's ear canal LEGOs. Let's go get a soda."

We hissed our bottles open and took a seat in the first-floor dialysis atrium—a bustling thoroughfare on weekdays but a bastion of calm on that predawn Saturday. We sipped in silence, eyes on the vista of Detroit in the dying night through a residue-speckled wall of windows. Orange soda and a Dr Pepper. Never too early or too late in the day for sugar and bubbles.

"How you feeling?" I ventured.

Lorisa cocked her head, eyes on the horizon.

"I mean, pretty terrible."

"Yeah. This was your first one?"

"Weirdly, no. I mean, I've had plenty of patients who've died on me before, but this one . . ." She took another swig and rolled her head in a long-overdue stretch. "This one, man . . ."

"First one that truly feels like it's yours."

"Exactly. First one where I'm drowning in the what-if's, you know?"

I did know.

"What if I'd gotten there sooner? What if I'd known the right way to hold pressure? What if I'd taken better charge of what was going on in the room?

"What if I'd just been better?" She sipped her Dr Pepper.

"I remember my first real one. Her name was Luz. And the way she died was just as bloody and traumatic and what-iffy, and I was just . . . Yeah, I was already in a pretty dark place. And that moment nearly pushed me over whatever edge I was dangling on."

We sat in silence once again. Somewhere in a nearby hallway a broom swept over linoleum, an elevator chimed its arrival, and footsteps echoed through dimly lit halls. The hospital was just opening its eyes to greet a new day.

"I guess it just makes me scared, you know? Feeling this way," said Lorisa, eyes on the ceiling's peeling paint. "Like, the guilt, the fucking sadness. I mean, that dude just *died*. It was messy. It was undignified. And I feel it. I feel his death in my *chest*. How am I supposed to keep going if I let moments like this affect me so much?"

I nodded. Took another sip of orange soda. I knew this question. I just didn't know the answer. But I gave it a shot.

"Well, I'll tell you, you *can* keep going. You just have to decide how you want to do it. And there's no right answer. Some folks choose to feel every death, every bad outcome. Others choose to shut the door on the pain and not even look at it. Both choices are right. There are amazing doctors from both sides of the coin.

"Personally, I'm a feeler. I always thought that letting in all of the feelings that come with all of these moments would keep me connected and make me better at my job. But man, that's a hard road."

I swirled my bottle as years of moments danced before my eyes. Moments both inside and outside the hospital's doors.

"The more I let in, the harder it was to hold, you know? There was never a break, never enough sleep, just on to the next tragedy until I just had nothing left. I tried so hard to feel everything that I ended up not feeling anything."

"And that's what I'm afraid of," said Lorisa. "'Cause I'm a feeler too. I think it's just how I'm wired. And the idea that allowing the hard shit in will chip away at me until I'm unrecognizable is fucking terrifying."

"It sure is."

"So what did you do?"

I sucked down the last splash of soda and closed my eyes.

"This. These moments." I looked out on the bare tree branches on the boulevard, frozen in the last moments of another winter's night. "We're in this job where every minute of the day, everyone in the world tells us how selfless we need to be. We are noble. We are the best of us, because we chose a job where we put other people first. So we internalize that. And in my opinion, that is the most toxic shit of all time.

"*You* are your most valuable possession. *Your* mind. *Your* health. *Your fucking sanity.* Put your fucking life jacket on first. If you don't and you try to save someone flailing in the ocean, what happens?"

Lorisa smiled. "You both fucking drown."

"You *both* fucking drown. So my advice? Force yourself to stop. I promise you there is always, *always* time to stop. Feel it all. Cry if you must. Learn what you can. Then turn the release valve, and let the rest go.

"However you choose to do it, you can make it through if you don't forget yourself. It's the one thing you can't afford to lose."

Lorisa sat in the quiet for a moment, then smiled, pounded the last of her soda, and let out a righteous belch. I couldn't help but crack a smile myself.

"Gross," I said, "but I guess that's as good a place as any to start."

We laughed and sat a few minutes more, watching the Detroit skyline defrost in the first rays of sunlight.

NINE

EULOGY

So, I had the dream again.

The Vegas dream, where I wake up in a hotel room face-to-face with my father.

And despite all I've learned, all I've embraced, all I've let go of, and all the progress I thought I'd made, I woke up gasping. Sobbing. Violently. Out of control. A dizzying confluence of shame and anger, frustration and disappointment, helplessness and hopelessness, all flung me like a rag doll. It felt like falling. And drowning. And dying. All at once.

Until I swung my legs over the side of the bed and felt the solid floor beneath my feet. My breathing slowed. I dried my eyes and the room came into focus. I took stock of each set of muscles I held in buzzing tension and released them one by one, just as I'd been practicing for the last few years. Toes, calves, thighs, hips, lower back, upper back, fingers, shoulders, neck, face. Then a deep, deep breath. And let it out.

Fuck. I thought I'd beaten this thing.

I don't know if the massive response that this dream still elicits is something to be beaten.

You're right. So many years of fighting and it always seems to win.

Maybe I've been hearing it wrong all this time. Seeing nothing but the obvious. It might finally be time to—

Understand.

I think I've grown enough to give myself a real chance. Where to begin?

How about at the beginning? The very first time. That night in—

Las Vegas.

It was my first trip to the city of sin. A family vacation with my mom and younger brothers. I was twenty-one, fresh out of college, and itching for ways to cement my transition into adulthood. So I tried gambling for the first time. It had always been a family taboo despite the brazen casualness with which my father had engaged in it daily. So on the flight to the desert, I'd resolved to not only see what the fuss was about but do it better than he did. Smarter. More responsibly. My game would be blackjack. The house odds were lower than the slots. There was skill involved. If I learned the rules, I stood a chance at being successful. I'd have much more control over my fate than in the gambling on horse racing he loved so much. And I gave myself a spending limit. That was key. Two hundred dollars. Nothing more.

If I ever felt my mind slipping into temptation, I'd remind myself that these were just games. Vegas wasn't a bogeyman to be feared. It was a playground masquerading as a city. There were millions of people who could play and not ruin their lives. Why not me?

So I played. And I won. And I kept winning.

Forty dollars turned into six hundred dollars. Then nine hundred dollars. As the minutes wore on and my pile of chips grew, a curious transformation took place: Tony, or at least the recognizable pieces of Tony, slipped away. I became anonymous even to myself as a baser, primal lust took over. Every hand dealt was foreplay, every card the dealer flipped a passionate thrust until that final card's climax when, for better or worse, it was over. I'd place another bet, sip another free cocktail, then start again. And again. And again.

I don't know where I went in those hours at the blackjack table, but I was awash with a discomfiting ecstasy that I'd never expected or experienced. I was powerful and powerless all at once. Dull warning bells sounded through my mind all night, alerting me to danger. But the danger made it intoxicating. Irresistible.

A glance at my phone brought me back to myself: 4:00 a.m. I'd been rooted to the same spot for six hours, lubricated by free drinks, fellated by a card game. *I should get to bed*, I thought to myself. *We're leaving to see the Grand Canyon in three hours*. But at that point, did I really need sleep? We were on vacation, after all. What was a couple more minutes? A few more hands? Maybe until I'd finished this drink. If I was going to leave, should I just bet it all on this last hand? Goddamn, what if . . . just what if?

Thankfully, *what if* lost the battle that night. Barely. My mind screamed in agony as I stepped away from the table. It was all I could do to put one reluctant foot ahead of the other. My pulse quickened. Tears came to my eyes. Pain was everywhere and nowhere, searing and silent. But I kept moving.

I made it to bed, my family's quiet snores all around me, and the revolt within slowly subsided, granting me sleep.

I had only one dream.

I woke to find my mother and brothers gone. Sunlight spilled into the room, defying the desert-grade window tints. Though I lay above the covers, the bedsheets had already been made neatly beneath my body. I sat up. The room was pristine. No luggage, no dirty clothes, no trace of anyone's overnight stay. The light was too bright. I had to shut the blinds. I turned to find a figure silhouetted, sitting at attention in perfect profile. A man. Waiting. Welcoming? I wasn't sure, but it felt right. I took the seat opposite him, straining to see his face for the first time.

It was my father. I almost didn't recognize him without his glasses, but there he was, appraising me with inscrutable eyes.

Somehow I'd been expecting him. I knew we'd be here sooner or later.

His lips turned up into the slightest hint of a smile.

And suddenly I was rooted to my chair. My muscles went rigid, locking me in place. My eyes struggled to escape his gaze, but it was impossible. He filled my vision. Only him. He shouldn't have been able to see more than four inches from his face without his glasses, but on that morning I knew he saw me clearly.

And there was nothing more terrifying in the world than that.

I couldn't breathe.

But I did scream. Air burned as my last breaths escaped me in roars of agony. Of fear. Of recognition.

I was going to die.

He smiled ever wider as my cries shook my body, filling every corner of the room with anguish.

As the last of the searing air passed my vocal cords and the final tortured croaks escaped my throat, my final thought was that there was no escape.

I was going to die there. With him.

Unmasked. Smiling his approval.

I woke up.

For the last ten years, the dream has hunted me—every ray of sunlight and reverberating scream and welcoming, beckoning crease of his face the same each time. And it always manages to find me in the moments where I've fallen suddenly, incurably lonely.

Is today one of those moments?

It's Father's Day.

Oh, of course.

Of course.

We used to talk on the phone every now and then. Even after he'd admitted to me he was a failure back when I was in medical school, he'd check in on occasion. At some point we began a passive war of communication attrition. He stopped calling to see how I was doing, so I stopped trying to find time to call him. One year he didn't call for Christmas, the next I didn't call for Thanksgiving. One year it seemed he'd discovered text messaging and sent one to me in lieu of a phone call on my birthday. I texted him on his birthday months later and heard nothing back. Last year I didn't hear from him at all on my birthday. Or Thanksgiving. Or Christmas.

So this year I decided not to reach out to him on Father's Day.

Primarily it was an act of self-preservation: continuing to treat our relationship as something that I had to maintain only out of obligation to my family had been wilting me for years. Reaching out to him (or waiting for him) only ever pushed me to try to understand him more: What was going on in his mind or his life or his other family that made him choose to ignore me? Or forget about me? Or see me as a stranger?

The answers never came. And his deepening silence only served to convince me that only one of us was even asking these questions.

I knew I'd never understand him. So I had to stop trying.

I had to stop calling. To save myself.

And yet.

Today—Father's Day—I wept. Through weary red eyes and depleted, shaking muscles. Because he didn't call me with disappointment. Or anger. Because my absence from his life didn't even warrant a response.

Because no matter what I accomplish in my life or who I become, no matter how faithfully I demonstrate his traits or how defiantly I strive to embody the opposite, no matter what, I'm never important enough to him.

He doesn't want me.

And that truth hit me in the gut full force today, doubling me over. The tears that fell today were tears of grief. Of mourning.

It's okay to feel all of that, and it's especially powerful to distill it down to that last word: mourning.

Power in mourning. I hadn't considered that.

There is power in every word you honestly express. I <u>know</u> you've recognized that by now. Over the last few years you've managed to change your entire world, the way you view yourself, the ways in which you wield your voice, and it all started <u>right fucking here</u>. By writing down the words that matter, no matter how hard they were to find. Even if you were the only one who'd ever read them, in them you found perspective. Confidence. Control.

And despite all of that, the one person who still has the power to rob you of—

Agency is him. Always, always him. He's the only thing in my life that still renders me voiceless. And small. Powerless and scared.

Thirty-plus years and he still has the power to revert me to childhood.

Fuck. That. Shit.

Fuck it indeed. Remember how you'd always whisper to yourself that it would—

All be easier if he were dead. The lifetime of wounds I received from him might dry up and scar over, instead of finding new ways to bleed whenever he walked back into my life.

Well, he may not be dead. But you can still lay him to rest.

A eulogy.

Not for him, but for the pieces of us that need letting go.

Not for him. For—

You and me.

So.

What will your words lay to rest, dead and buried?

I'll start with the death of what I've always known to be inevitable: the immutable conviction that all of his mistakes live within me, and that I'm destined to repeat them.

Looking back, I still find myself amazed by the power of this idea and all that it's begotten. If I'm honest, it's at the core of why I became a doctor. I didn't get into this to help people, or whatever I told them in the interviews. I was drawn to medicine because of its fundamental dichotomy—altruistic and masochistic in equal measure. The idea of being selfless for a living called out to me because running away from myself, being *less* myself, was all I ever wanted. And the knowledge that the road through medicine, through surgery, through *specialized* ENT surgery, would be grueling and merciless held its own allure. Because punishment and pain were what I felt I deserved.

I found a life in which I could destroy who I was every day. Find new ways to reinforce how much I hated myself every day. And continue waking up to a world that rewarded me for staying that way.

I did it all because I was the walking embodiment of all his shortcomings, weaknesses, missteps, and misdeeds.

But it's time that I accept explicitly, through these words that have taken me years to find, that there is no truth in my old understanding of myself.

I've already proved it.

I used to know that I'd never be able to defeat depression, just as he never did. All of the ways in which it shapes a life—its ability to magnify doubt and loneliness, intrude on thoughts with self-hate speech, call for self-harm and death—were givens for me. My faulty brain wiring.

But I did what he couldn't.

I found the power in naming it. Respecting it. Understanding my brain's tendency toward it so that I could navigate life alongside it. I take medicine every day now. Dosage fine-tuned. And I've found a therapist because, despite what my residency training had tried to teach me, mental health crumbles in isolation. Help is nothing to be ashamed of. And it helps the medicine work better.

I've learned my depression's triggers: looming tests and evaluations, ends of relationships, isolation, major life milestones, and changes in scenery. I've learned my depression's footsteps: procrastination, late nights awake, upticks in alcohol consumption, and the sudden urge to run away.

I know this mental illness now. It is a partner to me in this life. And that's okay. As long as I center myself enough to recognize what might wake it from sleep and its voice as it approaches, I'll know when to truly listen to my depression. We'll converse meaningfully and navigate anxiety and pain together so that it doesn't feel the need to rip the steering wheel from my grip. And if it does? I've got professional help at my fingertips to keep me safely on the road.

My father never learned this. But I did.

I used to know that addiction would take me sooner or later, just as it took him. Once I heard the siren call of my vices that night at the blackjack table, I figured it was just a matter of time before I succumbed. Maybe it would be gambling. Maybe it would be drink. Maybe it would be drugs. I was resigned to the idea that at least one of them would destroy me, so I figured I might as well find out which one and get it over with. For a long time, I thought it would be alcohol. I've leaned on it like a crutch for several years, craving its invitation to escape and hide and forget.

I waited for the tickle of dependence. In certain moments, I even hoped for it—pleaded with the bottle to take the choice out of my hands and relieve me of control over my cursed future. But it never did. My body didn't need it. My brain could function without it. When I wanted to, I could let it go without fear of my world collapsing. It was unhealthy substance use, sure, but it wasn't addiction. And although biology can play a strong role in whether the vulnerability to the illness gets passed down, I am, despite my most destructive efforts, miraculously one of the lucky ones.

I've been able to walk away from the blackjack tables.

He never could.

I used to know that I wasn't worthy of receiving real, lasting love, just as he felt he wasn't. But I learned after many seasons with a woman named Z that none of us are destined for heartbreak from birth. She taught me, painfully, that we all tend to bring around us the relationships we think we deserve. In the years that we both wallowed in despair and doubt and worthlessness, we were perfect for each other. Abuse was all either of us felt we were worth. It was all love could mean to us at the time.

And then we began our journeys of healing. Independent of each other, we did the work of probing ourselves for joy and peace and purpose. She moved on quickly. Got married. Although I felt the sting of losing her in the days after we let each other go, I was well on my way to discovering parts of myself that I loved and appreciated in her wake. We fell out of sync as our journeys diverged. We couldn't find the desperate electricity that had once linked us—even as a springboard for friendship—as neither of us was desperate anymore.

We both found that we deserved something different from love. Something other than each other.

What that will ultimately look like for me I don't know. But now that I recognize that my mind, my passions, my weaknesses, and my swirling pool of ever-changing feelings are worth caring for, protecting, and even sharing, I can finally believe that a partner who radically accepts and appreciates themselves may actually find their way into my life.

I used to know that I'd never become a father I could be proud of, that I'd never have the ability to put my own interests aside so that I could put the welfare of another first, just as he couldn't. But I survived residency long enough to become a chief resident. I was given the responsibility of leading my peers. I had a say in their success. It was an opportunity to wield a modicum of power in a fucked-up system, and all I could ever think about was how to pass that power on to those coming up behind me who had none. I pushed them, expected more of them than was expected of me at their stage. I listened to them, did all I could to embrace and respect their humanity and insecurities and disparate life paths and perspectives in a way that nobody had for me. I protected them, took criticism and anger and bullshit from the bosses on my own shoulders, so as to preserve their confidence.

Sometimes I did right by them, as I hope Jazlyn and Lorisa would attest. Sometimes I missed the mark, as I'm sure Waldo believes. But I was always there. I kept on showing up. Never ran away. Always managed to find the room for both my life and theirs.

I've got to believe that, at its most fundamental, that's what parenting is.

How can I go on fearing it when I already understand, have already lived what my father couldn't?

It's funny, I can barely write the words anymore, but for the sake of honoring the dead:

I am inevitably my father's mistakes.

That certainty, that indisputable truth, dies today.

How does it feel to let that go?

It feels . . . like a start? I can see now that there should be one last subject of this eulogy.

The pieces of him that I didn't run from—the ones I absorbed and even embraced—have always felt like poison to me. And they have, by and large, been what he understood to be the pieces that make up a man.

Keep your hair cut short and modest. Iron your pants. Start letting go of childish things as soon as you learn to talk. Use your brains to make money. Money means status and respect. But not safety. The world is full of those who don't deserve your trust. Especially women. Trust isn't what they're here for. Women are to be lusted over. To be vessels for your kids. To be agreeable ornaments. To be used as tools in whatever way you need them to be. Women are things. You don't need to listen to them. You don't need to answer their questions. Your secrets are your own. You don't owe them to anyone. Keeping your own counsel is how you show you're strong. And you have to be strong because of white people. White people run the world. And will never accept you. But in order for you to survive, they need to like you. So don't scare them. Keep your hair cut short and modest. Iron your pants. Start letting go of childish things . . .

I internalized it all. Believed it all to be true. Until my teenage years, when he made himself more and more scarce. In his absence, I began to question everything about him: his ability to tell the truth, the veracity of the lessons he'd taught me. Suddenly everything he believed about manhood seemed so farcical, so completely over the top in its inaccuracy, that all I wanted to do was reject it. I knew it was all wrong, but I knew of no alternatives, had no idea what was *right*. So despite my attempts to dispel them, his guiding principles continued to live within me. Influencing me. Guiding me. Disgusting me.

I hated all of the parts of myself that sprang from his masculinity lessons. And they were many.

It's taken nearly twenty years of war with myself, but only now, after having spent a lifetime performing for the world and hoping they'd see exactly what they wanted to see, can I finally see the truth behind his view of manhood. Being a man, according to my father, had little to do with who he was and everything to do with how he needed to be *seen*. His modus operandi was guided by his perceived weakness and sense of inadequacy, the assured knowledge that his value had been calculated by the world and had been found to be minuscule. So being a man was all about finding control in a world that he couldn't control. It was about begging acceptance from a world that dismissed him, ignored him, and thought he'd be better off dead.

But unlike him, I started writing. I woke up one morning years ago desperately compelled to find control and balance inside my head, while outside of it my world swirled in chaos. And in this pursuit I found a deceptively simple truth: my identity and my place in the world are determined by *me*.

My opinion of myself.

My *love* for myself.

And no one else's.

Becoming a man required an arduous realization of my own confident identity and strength of character. An embrace of my vulnerability. My sensitivity and kindness. And, perhaps above all, acceptance. Acceptance of myself and all of my complexities with curiosity and grace.

And ultimately, the humility and generosity to extend each of these gifts to the world around me.

To me, that's what it means to be fully realized.

And (surprise, surprise) these simple goals are *ungendered*. At their cores, what are manhood and womanhood but social creations that limit, stigmatize, and marginalize all that we are and can be? It took my father's struggles through manhood's trappings and his fractured and incomplete attempts at passing them on for me to realize that manhood was never the goal at all. Man, woman, boy, girl, and everyone in between; raised by the love of two parents, or just one, or none—identity and heart and beauty and greatness and truth are not, were never, at the mercy of the world but within us to build and love and shine. And that's pretty fucking dope.

So the truth that I held on to for so long—that the pieces of him that live in me are, and have only ever been, malignant and corrupting and worthy of nothing but contempt, shame, and hatred—must die today. In laying it to rest I realize that his gifts to me, flawed though they may have been, ultimately allowed me to evolve into something greater than my beginnings. They were the seeds from which a new perspective on "being a man" grew.

With all that said, I guess being born his namesake, living with the constant reminder of his contributions to who I am and where I come from, might have been the most valuable thing to ever happen to me.

What a mind fuck.

So what does that mean for me?

Where do I *go from here?*

Well, I've spent most of my life afraid to plan for a future. A consequence of not liking myself. The road ahead always seemed to be paved with mistakes of my own making. Too scary a sight. So I allowed myself to look only one step, one day, one hour ahead.

But now . . .

This tragic profession has taught me a great many things. Chief among them is the understanding that death and dying can beget new life. Over the course of my medical lifetime, I've seen the many faces of suffering and the many shapes of death countless times—in the eyes and last heaving breaths of patients, in the demise of my relationships with loved ones, and, of course, within myself. Without the unique trials of this journey, I'd have never experienced the death of my ego, my confidence, my defenses, and my compassion and kindness. And though I fall short of feeling grateful for medicine's ruthless path of destruction, I do find myself compelled to show appreciation. So much of me needed to die in order to make room for a new framework of life, and medical training provided a hellish, traumatizing context in which that transition could unfold. I might never have found the strength to navigate and ultimately celebrate the death of my most deep-seated roadblocks to happiness if not for the years of death practice I received in the hospital.

But now I feel that it's time for me to let medicine go.

I've done the work. Completed residency. Even passed one final eight-hour test and achieved the title of board-certified otolaryngologist. Got the certificate in the mail. It was shiny. And now I work every day in a private practice. And it's . . . fine. Everything's fine—the hours, the patients, the colleagues, the operations, the low emotional stakes—nothing truly worth complaining about. But the long days have managed to feel empty somehow. And the emptiness makes me restless.

I've been writing a lot these days. Telling stories, building characters and worlds. I've been letting music take me away, singing loudly in the shower and dancing naked in the mirror. Colors in nature arrest me. My photographs seem to capture the world's motion and momentum. I've even been crying in movie theaters—not the tears of repressed trauma but for the beauty of evocative storytelling.

Something has awakened inside me. Medicine got me here, but I don't love it. It doesn't sustain me. It never did. And I think that's okay. But a future built upon what I can create, especially with words—those same words that used to torment me with their elusiveness—sure feels like a future I could love.

The potential for a life of professional true love. It's enough to pull me through these empty clinic days. In my mind, I've already quit this bitch. New unplanned and unwritten adventures await.

And speaking of true love, I finally feel strong enough to dream of a future in which I find it in another. I'll know her by the way she demands that I face the world maskless; the way in which we fearlessly dream together; the curiosity and understanding we hold for each other's pasts, and the assurance that those pasts do not enslave our futures.

One day I'll meet her at the end of the aisle. We will speak loving commitments to each other with our whole hearts. Neither of us would be there if we hadn't done the difficult work of finding certainty. We'll surround ourselves with family we've chosen: the price of admission a promise to always lift us up—to support and bolster our union, our family, through the trials that will surely come. I'll hold no more fear of promises. I know now that they can be made for keeping, and not only exist for inevitable breaking.

And finally, the day of miracles will arrive and a new life will gaze upon me, cradled in the crook of my arm. If she's anything like me, her eyes will have questions from the moment they open. His little voice will hold power but he will search for direction. The echoes of my greatest fear—failure of fatherhood—will sing in my mind, answered by a vow from my heart to guide that little life with every scrap of wisdom I can muster, from that first moment through every one that follows.

Together we'll discover family. I'll show her that it begins as a nest, a place to observe and study the world before leaping. But someday she'll jump, and the strength of the family she was given will be measured by the quality of the family she chooses. A tall order, no mistake. Joy and folly will pepper her path as she evolves and discovers humanity in all of its complexity. I just hope she never forgets that she can always find a home in her mother and father when it's time to rest.

I'll show him that pain, in all of its forms, will come inevitably. This world can be angry, and unfair, and confusing, and cruel. The wounds may cut so deep that he'll fear what awaits when the blood finally runs dry. And if he's anything like me, his emotions will be too big for the number of words he knows to describe them. So I will be there to feel them right alongside him. Tears will fall. Anger will release. Disappointments and betrayals will feel as if they can cut him down. But I'll hold him close through it all. Together we'll embrace the pain in order to learn a new type of strength, a special kind of courage that would never have been found if we'd fled those feelings. He'll never face his emotions alone. And we'll allow ourselves the grace of knowing that the words will come later.

And what of madness? What if my chemical brain imbalances pass down to her just as easily as her smile and her eyes? Well, as long as I am here, she'll know that her mind is neither a curse nor a prison. Together we'll conquer the voices and name the foreign emotions as they arrive uninvited. We will discover the beautiful mysteries that reside in her mind right alongside the challenges. She'll never be handicapped. Because she'll know that her brain is wired just as it should be.

And love. He will know it from the moment he first cries out. He'll watch as his parents love each other through both doe-eyed, playful affection and the thankless, menial acts of understanding that each new day requires. Love will never be a trophy to covet or a currency that can be taken away just as easily as it is given—he'll receive it freely. Because all he ever had to do to earn it was emerge into this world.

"But how do I love myself?" he'll one day ask.

"Do you love yourself, Daddy?"

And with that, my little one will give me pause. I'll pull that little life into my chest and allow myself a moment to be overwhelmed. This child will be my dream, all of my dreams, made manifest. And he should know. She should know.

Should know all that it's cost me to learn to believe in dreams at all.

"I do," I'll begin. "I didn't always, but I learned."

"How?"

And I'll tell the full story. Out loud for the first time. The story of how I was scared to grow up because I didn't know how. The person who was supposed to show me the way was a grown-up who'd never learned how to grow up. He hurt my feelings every day and had no idea he was doing it because his mind was confused and sick.

He never loved himself. So he could never teach me what love was. But I knew I could learn.

I learned to love being exceptional and humble; angry and righteous; Black and visible; dark and witty; crazy and sublime; brilliant and shining.

Weird.

Imperfect.

Every last piece.

"Do you still love your daddy, even though he couldn't teach you?"

And the admission will finally come: In order to start loving myself, I had to stop loving him. Had to stop trying to understand him and asking why. I had to let my father go.

It still makes me sad. I mourn losing my love for him every day.

But I do thank him. Because I became who I am in large part due to who he was.

And I love myself a whole lot.

I'll run my hand through my little one's hair that night as we welcome bedtime.

"How will I know when I love myself? What does it feel like?"

And the words will fall from my mouth with hard-earned ease. So easily that I won't be able to help but smile in gratitude for the pain. For the journey. For my wings. For this life.

"Freedom. It feels like freedom."

So how was that?

Death and new *life, gratitude and* forgiveness, hopes and *dreams, love* and a *future. I'd say* I feel

Complete.

Like I might just have *embraced* this life.

And when *I lay* my *hea*d down to sleep tonight, and every night to come,

I can finally

*fi*nally

rest in peace.

Acknowledgments

This one goes out to so, so, so very many.

To my dream makers: First, my literary agent extraordinaire, Jon Michael Darga of Aevitas Creative Management. Thank you for being the first to take a chance on this story. Your enthusiasm from the start was infectious, and it bolstered my confidence when I needed it most. You're a pal and a confidant. Next, my brilliant editor, the mysterious Jake Morrissey of Riverhead Books. Thank you for seeing the potential of this book in its earliest iterations, and for pushing me to dig deeper at every turn. My journey through the seven stages of editorial grief were necessary to make this thing all it could be. Also, Rachel Christmas Derrick of Words Rule! Communications—I can't thank you enough for being my first professional reader, and for helping me understand what my story was truly about. Finally, big shouts to every single person who helped bring this book to life at both Aevitas and Riverhead. Though it took a long time to get here, the publishing journey has been a dream as a result of your hard work.

To my residency fam: Even here I won't drop your names, but you clowns know who you are. Though we all ended up moderately mutilated by the years of training, it was a pleasure growing up alongside you. I hope I was able to give voice to some of the things we felt too ashamed to share with one another.

To the fantastic women in medicine who lifted me up along the way: Dr. M! Little bro done grown up, huh? I don't think I've ever properly articulated this, but your belief in the type of doctor I was meant to be pushed me further than you might have ever imagined. I hope I didn't embarrass you. And of course, the Boss. Thank you for your support and belief in me as I limped over the finish line and beyond. You saw something in me along the way that made you decide that a lifetime investment in me was a safe bet. I won't let you down.

To my nonmedical Detroit family: You each had a hand in saving my life. I'll never stop being grateful for each one of you.

To my lifelong childhood friends: Anne, HaeNa, Jordan, Che, and Moosh. We did pretty well for ourselves, didn't we? Knowing you all have always been a call or text away since we were twelve years old has been a tremendous gift.

To my teachers: Ms. Pressman, thank you for sparking my true love of the stage. And for that day in high school when you knew I just needed to cry on your shoulder. Mr. Fennell, I went from being your B+/A− student to your friend and doctor. Rest peacefully, old man.

To Zach and Hank: I'm infinitely grateful that we rekindled and deepened our friendship when we did. It was right on time and fed me when I didn't even realize I was hungry. Zach, man, I miss you on most days. Thank you for continuing to smile, laugh, and demand the best of me from beyond the horizon.

To Dr. Zamudio: Thank you for helping me tap into the parts of myself that were nameless and voiceless for far too long.

To Katie: Thank you for being my first reader, my critic and cheerleader, my partner, my best friend, and my favorite person. I never imagined loving someone could be easy. Then you came along.

To my mother and brothers: Thank you for always giving me a place to call home, no matter how far my road has taken me. I hope I make you all proud.

And finally, to my father. It's taken me a lifetime to find these words to be true: Thank you, wherever you are. For all of it.